THE MEDICAL AND HEALTH CARE OF WOMEN

THE MEDICAL AND HEALTH CARE OF WOMEN

(A Sociological Study of Rural and Tribal Hilly Areas in Uttaranchal Pradesh)

DR. SWARN LATA SAKHUJA

GYAN PUBLISHING HOUSE

NEW DELHI-110002

The publication of this book has been financially supported by the Indian Council of Historical Research. The Responsibility for the facts stated or opinions expressed is entirely of the author and not of the Council.

The Medical and Health Care of Women : A Sociological Study of Rural and Tribal Hilly Areas in Uttaranchal Pradesh

ISBN: 81-212-0999-4

Published in 2008 in India by
Gyan Publishing House
5, Ansari Road, Darya Ganj,
New Delhi-110002
Phones : 23282060, 23261060
Fax : 011-23285914
E-mail: books@gyanbooks.com
Website: www.gyanbooks.com

Lasser Type Setting by: Rudra Computer Graphics, Delhi
Printed at : Singhal Print Media, Delhi

Contents

Foreword

Since last few decades, researches on various issues related to woman, such as marriage, family, education, inequality, exploitation etc. received vast importance among the scholars of various social sciences. Dr. Swarn Lata has chosen a major problem related to woman folk i.e. the Health Care of Women Living in Tribal and Hilly Areas of Uttarakhand. She has justified the importance of her subject in these words, "The issue of medical and health care of woman, especially her maternal health, is not important for woman herself only, but is the matter of major concern with the whole humanity, society and nation, because she is the mother of race, source of evolution, pivot of the family and the key agency of socialization of new generations of both the sexes who are the real wealth of the nation.

I appreciate her efforts to analyze the health problem in such a way that the reader of the book may get a whole reflection of strenuous life routine of the housewives of remote hilly villages of Uttarakhand. In concluding pages of the book, she has expressed her concern in these words 'due to culturally sanctioned secondary status of woman in family and society, triple burden of social roles i.e. reproductive, house hold chores and labour in production for earning money, coupled with hardships of hilly geographical situation of the region, most of the women of the rural and tribal areas of Uttarakhand were seemed more old than their actual age. Their pale and wrinkled faces, their weak and frail physique and bent backs, all these symptoms tell the story of ill health, poor economic condition, under-nourishment, inadequate quality of medical and health care during illness, time of pregnancy and child birth and over burdened labour of women living in the hilly regions.'

The concern, which the author of this book has expressed for rural and tribal women, is timely and considerable, I assure her that the B.J.P. Government of the state is planning to provide better medical and health facilities and every kind of welfare schemes for the betterment of child and mother in our state.

The author has developed women related concept of health in broader socio-cultural framework of society, so that the remedial efforts may be made in proper directions by the policy makers and government officials. Her work will be helpful for future researchers on the subject.

I wish Dr. Swarn Lata Sakhuja all success for future.

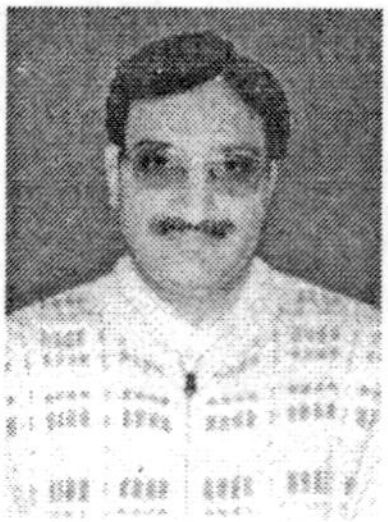

Dr. Ramesh Pokhrial 'Nishank'
Minister of Health & Education
Uattrakhand

Blessings

Health is a complex phenomenon for it involves elements of biology, culture and environment. Dr. Sakhuja's work on health care of women of rural and tribal hilly areas of Uttarakhand is a timely and effective study especially when women of this region make up more than half of the economically active population.

It goes without saying that deep knowledge of level of awareness, perception and cultural practices of health affecting behaviour among women is very important to make the ongoing health policies and programmes successful.

I congratulate Dr. Sakhuja for her sociological insight and depth to understand cultural dimensions of health and health seeking behaviour of the Uttarakhand women. Further researches will be all the more grateful to Dr. Sakhuja and her associates for this timely study.

I wish her great success for future.

A.R.N. Srivastava
Former Head of the Anthropology Department,
At present U.G.C. Emeritus Fellow,
University of Allahabad, Allahabad

Preface

Literary and historical researches show that gender discrimination has been a social reality from the very beginning of human civilization. It has been a disgusting paradox in the journey of cultural development of our civil society, that with the every stage of advancement, the status of women is going bad to worse in every sphere of social life. In the process of woman's degradation, half of the world's humanity had been deprived of its self respect, education, economic and political participation all over the world.

After independence, the Government of India granted several constitutional safeguard and statutory rights to women to elevate their status in family and society. But it is really unfortunate for the nation and society, that all these efforts remained only in the pages of constitution. The exploitation and deprivation in every sphere of life continued as ever. She is denied even the right to birth and life till recently. Woman of every stratum of society is facing innumerable problems in her day-to-day life even in this age of modernization and democratization.

There are numerous burning issues related to women which fascinate the students of social sciences and research scholars to know the reality hidden beneath the layers. The book in hand presents a sociological analysis of one of those myriad burning problems related to woman which is not important for woman only, but essentially, related to the existence of whole humanity, society and nation's life and the issue is 'the medical and health care of woman, specifically her maternal health.' Due to her anatomy and distinctive feminine qualities, the woman has been granted by nature, the boon of motherhood. She is the creator of whole of the humanity, source of evolution of human race, pivot of the family, key agency of socialization of new generations and of course the equal participant in the process of nation building in modern times. The entire range of activities related to human survival is performed by the woman, but the woman herself is the most neglected person in the family and society.

From above discussion it may fairly be understood that the health issue of woman is the matter of basic concern for any nation and society. The development, growth and prosperity of any nation depends on the health status of its citizens, especially on women's health because their health will determine the health and productivity of future generations of both the sexes, who are the real wealth of the nation.

In this book the author has adopted the interdisciplinary approach to reach the depth of the health problem, which means that every aspect of human's life is influenced and interconnected with the other aspects of life. While examining the health issue of women, the author has emphasized on the fact that health issue is not only a bio-medical phenomenon but it is a complex one, which is largely influenced by social and cultural factors which are deeply interwoven with the social fabric of life. In women's case the interrelationship between health and socio-cultural factors is more relevant as it is emphatically stated in the report of the Commission on the Status of Women in India (1974). "That for women, health is both an important factor in the achievement of status as well as the indicator of social status, because it is conditioned to a great extent by the social attitudes of society. These social factors also influence the provision and use of preventive and curative health care, including maternal care." C.S.W.I. report (1974). Thus the issue of medical and health care is the integral part of our socio-cultural system.

The subject matter of the book is based on a micro-field-study of some of the hilly and tribal areas of Uttarakhand State. In the effort to study the condition of health care of women, the author came to know that maternal health is a serious problem in India. The health care facilities provided by the government in the remote villages of hilly and tribal areas of the country are very much insufficient in quality and quantity both. Having briefly discussed the various aspects of health scenario of the country, with particular reference to rural and tribal villages of Uttarakhand, the author humbly suggested that the health care system of the country requires renewal, repair and reconstruction to make the health care system pro-poor, pro-rural and pro-underprivileged classes of the country, who are the real persons to get the benefits of public health care system.

The book also presents a bright side of social life of the people living in remote hilly areas of Uttarakhand. From field survey, the author observed that despite the poverty and deprivation of modern facilities of life, the villagers belong to a strong social support system, due to integrated interrelationship and warm emotional ties among the members within the community, they stand by each other in times of illness, child birth or any other emergency and even, they help each other financially also.

The book is an academic venture and purely empirical and exploratory sociological analysis, based on the facts obtained through schedules, observations and intensive interviews from the respondents (women) of Dehradun and Almora Districts of Uttarakhand State. The interpretation of facts on the basis of data; had been done as far as possible objectivity, subject to the constraint of human error.

However, a humble effort had been made to present the true picture of women's health hazards living in remote hilly areas, with the hope that the analysis and findings may be used for making proper health policies and programmes to elevate the health status of women.

Dr. Swarn Lata Sakhuja
Retired Reader
Deptt. of Sociology
M.L. & J.N.K. Girls (P.G.) College,
Saharanpur

Acknowledgements

The publication of this major research project was only possible with the constant moral support and co-operation of several persons and institutions.

I take this opportunity to express my deepest sense of gratitude to Professor A.M. Khan, I.C.S.S.R. consultant and Dr. Prem Prakash Pandey, Assistant Director I.C.S.S.R. New Delhi, who evaluated my research report very sincerely and very minutely. I am thankful to both of them for their recommendation to the survey and Publication Department of I.C.S.S.R., New Delhi to bear the cost of publication of this book.

I am thankful from deepest core of my heart to Honourable Minister, Dr. Ramesh Pokhrial (Nishank), Ministry of Health and Education, Uttarakhand State, who was kind enough to give his invaluable time for writing very inspiring foreword for my book, despite his busy schedule and ministerial responsibilities. Since Dr. Nishank is a literary person and an eminent scholar of many disciplines and also an "Ayurvedacharya" and a great promoter of public health programmes, that he not only appreciated my suggestions in this book but also promised to implement health policies and welfare programmes for rural women living in hazardous condition in the remote and distant areas of Uttarakhand.

I am heartily thankful to my teacher, Professor A.R.N. Srivastava, Former Head of the Anthropology Department, University of Allahabad, at present U.G.C. Emeritus Fellow, University of Allahabad, whose constant inspiration and guidance made possible the nascent beginning of this research work. I express my deepest gratitude for blessings which he expressed in his encouraging words for the book.

I am thankful to Dr. Nilanjana Kishore, Principal, M.L. & J.N.K. Girls P.G. College, Saharanpur, who had always encouraged me to undertake the major research project and co-operated me positively, at every step of official formality.

I am also thankful to my colleagues & friends. Mrs. Sudershan Gandhi, Dr. Madhu Jain, Dr. Surender Makkar, Dr. Padmaja Amit, Dr. Nirmal Dindra, M.L. & J.N.K. Girls P.G. College, Saharanpur for their valuable suggestions and co-operation for this work.

I also express my gratitude to Dr. K.D. Gaur, Deputy Director, I.C.S.S.R., New Delhi, who, on my request guided me in the initial stage of preparing the 'Project Proposal' during his official visit to our college, M.L.& J.N.K. Girls P.G. College, Saharanpur.

Further, thanks to all those officials and authorities of I.C.S.S.R., New Delhi, for providing me every kind of co-operation and financial assistance, necessary for making the task possible.

I have been benefited by the library facilities of S.N.D.T. (Mumbai), I.C.S.S.R. (Delhi) and M.L. & J.N.K.Girls P.G. College, Saharanpur. I thank to the personnels of these centres.

In humble words, I am thankful to Mrs. Kamla Panth, President Pragatisheel Mahila Manch, Dehradun and the Investigators of both the districts – Dehradun and Almora for their invaluable co-operation for field stury. At the same time, I am heartily thankful to all informants, including the personnels of P.H.Cs., M.H.Cs., Hospitas and N.G.Os., who after several persuasions, gave their positive co-operation. After all this work is the feelings of these people.

Last but not least, I thank Mr. Vineet Gupta, 'Ganpati Electrostat', Saharanpur for composing manuscript and designed an attractive cover page for the book.

- Dr. Swarn Lata Sakhuja

List of Tables

1

Introduction

Part I

Problem and Perspective

This research project presents a sociological analysis of one of the myriad burning issues related to womankind which is not important for the life and existence of woman herself only, but essentially, related to the existence of whole humanity, society and nation's life, and the issue is 'The Medical and Health Care of Women' with special reference to their 'Reproductive Health'.

The health issue of womenfolk, during last some decades, is gaining more and more concern with the scholars of various disciplines, specifically with the thinkers of demography, sociology, economics and medical science as well as with the pioneers of woman-studies and advocates of gender-justice and of course at the same time with national policy makers and government officials too. The reason behind this vast range of concern is that the health issue of women has multifaced repercussions on other important national issues, such as low and continuous declining proportion of women in India's population since 1901 census, high (female) infant mortality rate, increasing trend of female-foeticide, weak physique and low efficiency level of new generations, less participation of women labour-force in economic activities etc. and ultimately on the growth rate and the development process of the country at large. An issue, which has so many significant implications on the social life of the masses, it is but natural for a student of sociology to go deep into the subject and to enquire the ground reality beneath the layers. Thus the researcher has made an humble attempt to study the problem of medical and health care of women with the help of a micro-field-study of some of the hilly and tribal areas of Uttaranchal Pradesh.

Although, health is generally considered a bio-medical phenomenon, and illness and diseases are treated with bio-medical approach. But with the emergence of medical sociology and the modern humane approach to the health problems, it is vastly admitted and accepted that health of an individual or community is a complex phenomenon which is largely influenced by social and cultural factors which are deeply interwoven with the social fabric of life. Pokrana (1994) stated that "illness and disease are an outcome of macro-interactions of the bio-socio and environmental factors". Imboden, Canter, Cliff and Trevo (1961) also stated that "the cure of illness depends on cultural background and emotional conditions of a person"; Saunder (1954) also observed that "health and cure is related to age, sex, occupation, marital status etc. which indicate the social status of a person".

To study the health and sickness behaviour of a community, one may not get the full understanding of the problem in depth, unless one inquires the socio-cultural factors affecting the health care system, health related beliefs and practices, traditional and religious health care institutions, personal hygiene and life-style of the people etc. These are the areas in which social scientists have significant role to play not less than their medical counterparts, more-over it is better to say that the role of social-scientists is indispensable for better understanding and solving the health problems of the masses.

Madhu Nagla (1997) emphasized that medical care or the treatment of illness is not only a chemical and physical process. The cure of a patient is also concerned with his or her culture, personality, norms and values. The societal belief in a certain therapy, be it indigenous, traditional or cosmic, contributes substantially in his recovery.

The inter-relationship between illness and health and a given social situation is not entirely new to the field of sociology. Right from the pioneer social thinkers like Hippocrate, Durkheim, Ogburn, Spencer to modern social thinkers like Parsons, Wilson, Hawkins and others directly or indirectly stated illness and disease as a social phenomenon and suggested the social environment as an etiological factor in disease and illness and emphasized doctor-patient relationship as a therapeutic tool. Durkheim (1938) treated sickness as a state of deviation from normalcy. He observed that "sickness disturbs day-to-day routine. All societies have social mechanisms to deal with strains and conflicts that deviation of any kind inevitably creates". He described suicidal attitude as acute state of mental illness and established a cause effect relationship between suicide and social environment. He concluded that "it is because society, weak and disturbed lets too many persons escape to completely from its influence. Thus, the only remedy for the ill is to restore enough consistency to social group for them to obtain a firmer grip on the individual and for him to feel himself bound to them". Durkheim (1897), Talcott Parsons, the pioneer thinkers of modern social theory, treated sickness and disease as a pathological social phenomenon. In a series of papers from 1951 to 1958, Parsons developed his concept of 'Sick Role' and defined it as a form of deviance and described it as disturbance in the capacity of an individual for normally expected task or role performance, which is not specific to his commitments to any particular task, role, collectivity, norm or value. Parsons (1972) opined that "it is obligation of family members and related state agencies to help the sick person to get well".

Another, modern social thinker Freidson (1967) also described 'illness and disease' as 'social problem' and suggested that it should be dealt with the organizations or offices of social control. Morris (1973) also stated that notions of health and illness are influenced by complex inter-action between individuals, their socio-cultural settings and the physical environment.

No doubt disease or ill-health strains the whole social set-up i.e. cultural, technological, economic, political, legal and welfare systems of the society in which it occurs. For this reason, early thinkers of sociology described the state of ill-health as a pathological social phenomoenon and they tried to explore the remedial measures to eliminate this situation.

Prof. Swain, (1994) observed that the realization of multifactoral causation of disease process has brought the social and medical scientists close together to fight against the common enemy. Thus, it may be said as K.L. Pokrana and Singhi (1994) stated that "Certainly the study of medicine is neither new nor tangential to the field of sociology".

The entry of sociology in the field of health, disease and medicine is getting a rapid pace between 1946 and 1955 in U.S.A., chiefly among relatively young workers in Sociology, Anthropology, Social Psychology and Psychiatry and it was felt that a specialized branch of medical sociology should be developed. Albrecht and Higgins (1979) stated that as a specialized field, medical sociology encompasses a wide range of substantive areas; definitions of health and illness, etiology of morbidity and mortality, the social and cultural dimensions of health and illness, the social psychology of health and illness, medical personnels and their behaviour, and organization, delivery and polities of health care services.

Thus we see that health and social factors are inalienable to each other as observed by Pokrana (1994) "Health, illness and disease are significant dimensions of man and society. They are integral part of man's knowledge and existence. Sociological knowledge supplements and some times it helps to explain phenomena, causes of disease and possible solutions beyond what has been explained by medical knowledge." Keeping in view the close inter-relationship between health and society, S.R.Mehta (1987) stated that "Medical sociology as a discipline, has to develop and grow as an area within the general field of sociology."

It would not be out of context here to mention one more important point about health and disease that in the present century, the health issue of the people does not remain personal concern of an individual or his family, but it has become a public issue. Markandey Singh Yadava (1994) stated that "the world-vide effects of world wars Ist and IInd have forced the nations to rethink the health problem of the masses in broader perspective". The emergence of slums and labour-colonies and their unhygienic conditions on one hand and the problem of numerous injured, handicapped and mentally retarted generations of war victims on the other, have stirred the hearts of human-right pioneers, thinkers, social workers and social-scientists and intellectuals of every discipline. Many articles and editorials were written to high-light the issue. One great social survey was carried out by sir Edwin Chadviek in the field of public health and an elaborate report was published in 1942 titled "Sanitary Condition of the Labouring Population of Great Britain". Similarly in United States, Lemuel Shattuck (1948) collected extensive social survey data regarding health and published it. Karl Marx, the great soical thinker and an acute critique of capitalist society, lamented about the miserable conditions of factory workers and their consequences in terms of mortality and morbidity. The result of this kind of public awareness motivated the leading nations to activate policies in this direction. In 1948, Britain had passed the Public Health Act. After published survey report by L. Shattuck in United

States, an official public health agency was established. The Governments of Russia, Turkey, Yugoslovakia also made efforts for public health measures. In 1919, the then Government of India also enacted a Public Health Legislation. Thus the public health movement took a momentum world over. Since then it is admitted that the protection and development of good health of masses, particularly of the poor and the down-trodden is the liability of the government and community.

In the light of above discussion, it may fairly become justified that there is vast scope for the student of sociology to study the health problem of any social group, segment or community at large. Present endeavour, in the form of research Project took the courage to understand this complex social problem of women folk.

Now the question arises that what is the importance of health for a person ! The answer to this question could not be understood better than through that mythological episode described in the great epic 'Mahabharata', in which Yaksha asked the eldest Pandava brother Yudhishthira "लाभानामुत्तमं किं स्यात्" ? (What is the most precious thing in the world for human happiness ?) The wise Dharmraj Yudhishthira answered "लाभानाम् श्रेयः आरोग्यम्". (The most precious thing in the world for human happiness is a disease free healthy body with healthy mind.) Singhi and Pokrana (1994) also stated that, "in ancient Greece as well as in India health was conceived man's precious possession and was treated as a cherished goal of life."

This eternal truth had been essence of life from time immemorial. Every person on earth aspires a healthy long life with totally fit and healthy sense organs. In vedic age, great seers used to pray God :

" पश्येम् शरदः शतम्, जीवेम् शरदः शतम्
श्रणुयाम शरदः शतम्, प्रव्रमाम् शरदः शतम्
अदीनः स्याम शरदः शतम् भूयश्च शरदः शतात्"
यजुर्वेद 36/24

If health was realized, the most precious treasure of life in ancient age, it is as much precious in modern, scientific age as well. Eminent Economist Whipple observed that "A nation's true wealth is not in its land and waters, not in its flocks and herds, not in its treasure of dollars, but in its healthy and happy men, women and children." (Whipple 2001) Djurfeldt (1980) also stated that health status of the people is an indicator of the level of social, economic material and environmental development of any society. Health is the primary factor and foundation stone of human personality. The development, growth and prosperity of any society or nation depends on the health status of its citizens. Of course it is the health of women that will, to a large extent determine the health and productivity of future generations of both the sexes, who are the real wealth of a nation.

Here, it should be mentioned that although the specific purpose of this study is 'The Medical and Health Care of Women', and academically the study should be concentrated itself on women's health issue only, but for the student of sociology, it is impossible to alienate any human problem from its socio-cultural context and to study it in an absolute manner, specially of women's health which is totally the outcome of socio-cultural setup of any society, modern or traditional. So an humble attempt has been made for better understanding to analyze the health problem of women relative to the status and role of woman in family and society at large.

Women and Society

Literary and Historical researches show that in early periods of human civilization, gender discrimination was least observed, Marxian Anthropologist Eleaner Leacock stated that in pre-class societies sex-roles were reciprocal, women were highly autonomous and social structures were sexually egalitarian" (Mathew ans Nair 1986).

In ancient India too, the glorious traditions of vedic period granted equal opportunities to men and women almost in every sphere of social life.

But unfortunately, the decay of vedic traditions and several other drastic changes that took place in Indian society, led to the curtailment of the freedom of women. The actual decline in the status of women and corresponding consolidation of patriarchal authority, began during the age of Manusmriti and other Shastras and Sutras. The degradation of women's status to its last limit reached in Moghal period. Upto 19th century, half the worlds humanity had been deprived of its self-respect, education, economic and political participation all over the world.

During the independence movement of India some liberal thinkers and leaders were compassionately moved by the pitiable condition and the utter-degradation of women. They induced the masses and started the reform movements against the fatal customs regarding women. With the dawn of Independence, Indian Government adopted the pattern of Socialistic Democratic Welfare State by constitution based on the values of Justice, Liberty, Equality and Fraternity. The deprived, the downtrodden and the weaker sections of society were provided special safeguards through the directive principles of state policies as the integral part of constitution.

The constitution of India considers women also as a weaker section of society-deserving special protection, care and welfare. To fulfill this task, many constitutional measures and statutory rights were granted to women to elevate their status in family, society and in national life.

As a result of these measures and efforts, no doubt the status of women has undergone considerable change, but the fact remains as stated in the report of the Commission for the Status of Women in India (C.S.W.I. 1974) "It was felt by the government of India, that while these changes have been considerable in the urban areas, specially in middle and upper middle classes, the problems continued to remain virtually unchanged in most of the Rural Areas".

It is really unfortunate for the nation and society, that women resource, which constitute nearly 50 percent of the total Human Resource, has been deprived of its self respect, education, adequate medical care, health, food and nutrition, economic and political participation after 58 years of independence of the nation. She is denied even the right to birth and life till recently.

Although, demographically women constitute half of the humanity, but in the real sense, she is the creator of whole of the humanity. Woman is a unique individual force in the life of human being. Due to her anatomy and distinctive feminine qualities, nature has imposed on her the burden of gestation, parturition and lactation of the child, who is the source of evolution of human race. The bearing and rearing of the child is the whole sole responsibility of the mother. She is the main agency of socialization of new generations in the family or the household. A family, which is the basic unit of society, is nurtured and preserved by the woman. She is the pivot of this basic unit- 'the family' Maitrai Krishan Raj (1988) emphasized that the entire range of activities related to human survival such as "Cooking, cleaning, child care, care of the sick and elders, animal care, kitchen garden etc. are performed by the woman."

Besides, these indispensable duties, women of today from educated middle and upper-middle strata of society are making appreciable contribution in many intellectual, technical and professional fields of 'Nation Building'. More over in the present age of globalization, liberalization and acute materialism, economic prosperity and high standard of living is the ambition and urge of every one in society. Due to roaring price hike of present time, it is very difficult for the masses to maintain their household needs and the education of children single-handedly, only with the earning of the male. It has become the necessity that woman should share the financial burden along with performing the household duties.

Besides this, in many miserable circumstances such as in widowhood, divorce, drunkardness or joblessness of the husband, women have to play the role of breadwinner along with the rearing of children and other dependents of the household. So the women of every strata of society today are facing the stress and strain of role conflict and over-loaded labour. Of these the condition of poor class women living in slums, rural and tribal areas is too strenuous to be described. They are deprived of bare necessities of life and are vulnerable to face every kind of exploitation, although they make the major part of unorganized sector of labour force of the country.

Health and Women

In women's case the health issue is not merely a medical or physical phenomenon, but it is a complex social phenomenon. It is emphatically stated in the C.S.W.I. report (1974) "That for women, health is both an important factor in the achievement of status as well as the indicator of social status, because it is conditioned to a great extent by social attitudes of society. Society delineates women's role partly according to their biological functions and partly from prevailing attitudes regarding their physical and mental capacity. These social attitudes also influence the provision and use of preventive and curative health care, including maternal care." The Government's documents indicate that the health problems of women such as the higher maternal and infant mortality, maternal morbidity, lower expectation of life at birth, malnutrition, mental disorders, suicide rate and certain sex related diseases are linked to the status and role of women in society.

The relationship between the health care attitude and status of women in society is the integral part of our cultural system. Davis and Blake (1974) stated That "The cultural norms that particularly affect women's health are the attitude to marriage, age of marriage, the values attached to fertility and sex of the child, attitude to family planning and the ideal role demanded of the women within family organization and social conventions. They determine her place within the family, the degree of her access to medical care, education, nutrition etc."

The effect of Patriarchy system also has great influence on the medical and health care system on women. Dandekar and Kumudini (1957) found in their study of rural communities that "The percentage of males getting medical treatment was higher than females and even more adult women had to be content with free or traditional treatment or no treatment." The role of woman as mother and a housewife and care-taker of every person in the household is also linked with her low health status. In all the households in India, it is customary for woman to serve the family first and then to eat whatever is left, generally males eat first. Because of this custom, not only in poor families, but in well to do families too, women generally suffer from malnutrition and anemia.

After the survey of long three years period, 'The Commission on the Status of Women' reported that, "All the available evidence leads us to conclude that high female mortality rate and decreasing female ratio after every census is due to the consistent neglect of Female Health." (C.S.W) (1974, p 312).

From the above statement of C.S.W.I it has been obvious that, after independence, although the Government of India has made considerable efforts to initiate and implement the health policies for women and children, such as to formulate 'separate division' in planning commission for women and children, in 1978, "Health for All by 2000 AD", in 1983 to enact Comprehensive Health Policy which has enunciated the long term demographic goals and other selected time bound programmes to elevate the health status of masses. Besides these measures, significant achievements have been made in the production of Drugs, Vaccines, Hospital Equipments and trained medical personnels and specialized doctors and surgeons.

From the analysis of measures taken by the Government, a rosy picture of Health status of the country may be drawn. But if we compare the progress of health policies, programmes and their implementation in terms of the people's needs, the overall picture of rural areas, tribal areas and slums in the urban areas, remain dismal in the country. The Department of science and Technology has rightly observed that "There is mismatch in what we know and what we are able to do to combat, these diseases. To a great extent, this is related to socio-economic development and administrative capabilities of a given society."

Above all these facts, one major factor should also be mentioned here about the modern medical and health care system in the country, which has adverse effects on women's health care. The modern medical network has become very much costly which is beyond the reach of the poor classes of society. So in developing country like India, the modernization of medical facilities in public sector has demanded a heavy price from national economy. The rapid growth of population, specially in poor and backward classes, index go together. In poor households, women are the most neglected persons in matter of health, medical care and nutrition.

The result is inescapable from the above statement, discussion and description, that health services and facilities are not available to all areas, segments, classes and people according to their needs and expectations in the country. So there is vast gap between people's needs and facilities made available by the Government and other relevant agencies. The people living in below the poverty line make somewhat 40% of the total population of the country. Due to living in unhygienic conditions and malnutrition, the people of this section are more prone to diseases. Most of the epidemics affect this poorer sections of the population in very serious proportion which affects to health status and development process of the country. Because of poverty, backwardness and huge size, they require medical care correspondingly in more proportion from the Government resources, which are already insufficient in quantity and quality both.

So there seems to be a vicious-circle of poverty and health problem in the backward, down trodden and weaker sections of society vis a vis to national scenario. This complicated national problem needs to be tackled seriously.

As a remedial effort to lessen this major problems of the country, a committed class of Social scientists, Anthropologists and research oriented personnels can contribute a lot in generating relevant information of various micro-groups and communities or societies by scientific investigation. They may prepare data profile, may analyze reports and they may render valuable suggestions based on the felt needs of the people which may be very much useful for Policy makers, National Planners and other relevant agencies established by the Government for the task.

It is hoped that the analysis and the findings of the present study "The Medical And Health Care of Women" Living in 'Rural and Tribal Hilly Regions of Uttaranchal Pradesh', will make contribution in the realm of research and knowledge and also may be used for making proper policies and programmes to elevate the Health status of the vulnerable sections of society.

Part II

Review of Literature

The pioneering and independent studies on various aspects and problems of women's lives received vast importance in post independence era in India and after the world war II in countries abroad. The main focus of these studies was on the issues like inequality, injustice and oppression, which have been the sources of women's low status in society and secondary status in the family.

Some studies concentrated on such aspects of women's lives as marriage and family, education, exploitation of women, politics and religion etc. Some of them are on the issues like women's participation in the unskilled; skilled and professional jobs and their problems of role conflict.

A class of sociologists, educationists, Anthropologists and the scholars of medical science had written a lot in the field of medical and health in India and abroad. Research literature in the field of medical sociology and health continues to expand in the form of journals, periodicals and research based books in every civil society and nation today.

Here, a brief discussion and main findings of those researches, books and reports is presented which have been directly or indirectly found useful in the formulation of the hypotheses and in selecting the problem and area of the present study.

Studies Related to the Status of Women in Society

A.S. Altekar (1962) in his classic text on the status of 'Hindu Women from Prehistoric times to the Present day' analysed the status of upper-castes elitist section of women within the Aryan Vedic traditions. The study concluded with the notion that with the decay of vedic traditions the degradation of women started slowly and steadily which reached its last limit with the invasion of moghals in India.

Towards Equality : Report of the Committee on the Status of Women in India : (CSW) (1974) is a government's effort undertaken for the first time to assess the real position of women in India. The survey was conducted during the period 1971-1974. Starting with a new perspective, a team of researchers and scholars have collected a large body of data on different aspects of women's lives. It identified "unexpected trends in women's situation such as decline in sex ratio, declining economic participation rate and growing gaps in life expectancy and mortality rates between men and women (Unesco report,1983). Some chapters are very much useful and relevant for study in hand, mainly chapter VIII, part II, 'Health Programme for Women'. The report says that Health is both an important factor in achievement of status as well as an indicator of social status particularly for women, whose health is conditioned by social attitude of society more than her physical and mental capacity. The report analyzed the demographic trends and came to the conclusion that "All the available evidence leads us to conclude that high female mortality rate and decreasing female ratio after every census is due to the consistent neglect of female health".

'Women in India' by Neera Desai(1977) is a pioneering work on Indian women from feminist perspective. It examines the changing position of women in India in various historical epoch and found that although there seems a change in the status of women in terms of statutory rights and constitutional safeguards granted to women after independence, but some historical fundamental factors still prevail in Indian social milieu which affect the status of women in modern age to gain equality to men.

'Hindu Women : Normative Models' by Prabhati Mukherjee (1978) is an attempt to understand the normative structure governing woman in Hindu society. The study found that it has been the effort of Hindu Social System throughout the ages that women should be assigned status and role in such a way that patriarnchial ideological system may be preserved and persist.

'Symbols of Power' by Veena Majumdar (1978) presents the political status of women in India. The Study concluded that women have been granted formal political rights but quite a few of them are occupying positions of power. Gender injustice in political field is also the stark reality of the situation till today.

. Neera Desai and Vibhuti Patel (1985): in their 'Monograph' presented a countrywide report on the impact of ID for women. They critically reviewed the issues like demographic trends, health, employment, unemployment situation and socio cultural factors etc. They also critically evaluate and conclude that the policies and programmes of development for women's education, health and welfare are very much inadequate for women's needs.

Devki Jain and Nirmala Banerjee (1985) made a collection of Essays on Women in Poor Households. The Study emphasized that, there is need to remove the inequality in nutrition, in comparison to work load to maintain women's health.

Neera Dasai and Krishan Raj (1987) in their book presented an Interdisciplinary Feminist Perspective, which is very useful in understanding the status of women in India in its real sense, women's place in society, economy, in family, their education, health etc. are dealt in detail and in a very penetrating manner. The various forms of atrocities and violence against women have been presented with proof and data, which show that with the benefits of education and economic participation the status and condition of some middle and upper middle class women have been elevated to some extent, but the bulk of women is deprived of the benefits granted by the constitutional safe guards.

Studies Related to Health and Disease

Studies abroad

The trend regarding the study of health and sickness behaviour in the field of sociology made a start in European countries first. Rivers, W.H.R. (1924) studied the illness behaviour among tribal people and revealed that the primitive belief regarding sickness was related to supernatural powers. The cause and remedy both were guided by the spiritual experts in the state of disease.

Clements F.E. (1932), Ackrknehct, EH (1942, 1943) and Sigerist HE (1951) also studied the causes and the system of cure of diseases prevailed in primitive societies. They concluded that certain tribes have developed a system which logically explains the relationship between state of illness and religion, magic and supernatural powers.

Miner, H, (1956), Jarvise DC (1958) and Eaton J.W.(1958) have studied the traditional and folk medicine system of illness and treatment among several rural and tribal communities. They revealed that these systems develop naturally within the process of socialization of generations after generations and these are unquestionable elements which are followed and respected by every member of society. These behaviour patterns and systems of treatment persist because they had achieved the sanctions of whole community, specifically of elders and religious leaders.

Hassinger and McNamare (1988) have studied the relationship of the public with physician in a rural setting in Mississippi, Saunders and Bruening (1959) have described hospital-community relationship in Mississippi and found that hospital administration is the key to the hospital's community relations.

Hamed Ammar (1960), an Egyptian sociologist, studied some rural areas of Middle East and found that they believe that illness and disease come when one fails to perform religious rituals properly or the failure to give the promised offering to a saint.

Frank J.D. (1961), studied in Subanun Community and found that the disease and illness originate from depression, tension and frustration which are psychological emotions. In this community the treatment of disease is a part of their culture.

Newman PL (1964) has researched the disease behavior of New Guinea Highland community. He emphasized more on social and cultural factors of disease than biological. Ground, John. G (1964) has studied Kenya people and found that the main cause of illness among the community is malnutrition. He stated that 60 to 70 percent death of children under the age of 6 years is the result of under-nourishment and wrong nourishment.

Fabrega, H.J. and D Silver (1970) Netting R.M. (1973), Riessman (1974), Stevenson (1975) have studied respectively the health behaviour of Jinakentan Community, Kabyars of Nigeria, poverty, illiteracy, cultural norm and health behaviour of some tribes, Haide of Iceland. All these studies revealed that health behaviour of these communities is regulated by cultural, ethical, economic and the beliefs related to the souls of dead persons and concept of rebirth.

Milan (1974) Surveyed health conditions among Eskimos in South Western Alaska and observed that disease and extreme poverty go together side by side. He also studied the development of their contemporary health care system.

Dixon M (1979) briefly reviewed current research on health, nutrition and medicine in rural Alaska and recommended that Anthropologists have much to contribute to future health research including work as both consultants and of researchers.

Ford Ann.S. and Ford W. Scott, (1980) in their article in Social Welfare (Journal of Sociology) have emphasized on health education and health life style for the people of any community.

Kroeger, A, (1980) in his unique study analyzed the inter-relationship between the diseases like asthema and other breathing problem and housing condition such as the situation, building material, ventilation and size of house and number of inhabitants etc.

Studies in India

The knowledge and cure of health and illness related behaviour is not new in Indian society. The health and medical system in India is supposed to be originate 5000 BC in vedic age. The oldest medical systems which were popularly prevailed in India were Ayurved, Yoga, Charms and Magic (Tantra, Mantra and Sidhi Vayvastha). The oldest Indian Physician was a great scholar Guru Aatray who was a teacher in Takshshila University. His teachings and medical cure techniques were collected and compiled by 'Rishi Charak'. The compiled work is known as 'Charak Sanhita', which is great scientific source and inspiration for every medical research. Even in modern age of allopathic revolution, Ayurvedic and Yoga systems are very much popular, not in India only, but in western countries too.

No doubt, the knowledge and cure systems about diseases were available in Indian mythological literature in aboundon, but field studies and research work about health and illness behavior of the people of different communities were the rare concepts for Indian Scholars till the nineteen century.

Although the problem of health, sanitation, illiteracy and poverty in tribal and remote rural areas in India were very much serious but due to isolated geographical situation, these areas remain untouched and neglected by Indian researchers. In late nineteenth century and early 20th century some Christian Missionary Fathers made first attempt to reach these areas and contacted the people of these isolated and neglected regions. They started the 'work of mercy' for their upliftment. They were the first scholars who studied the health and illness problems and inquired their traditional methods of cure and treatment. In late 20th century the Indian anthropologists and other social scientists made some attempts in this field.

Father Bodding, PO, (1925) in his study 'The Santhal and disease' had analyzed the causes of disease and epidemics in Santhal tribe and found that there is great role of traditional 'Ojjhas' and specialists of religion and magic performers in the treatment of sick people. He also studied the orthodox beliefs and rituals regarding sickness and infirmity such as Santhals believe that coughs are caused by mist and fog, ophthalmia is held to be the result of bath in first rainfalls and so on.

Ishvaran, (1938) studied the assumptions about sickness in south Indian villages and found that there are five categories of illness and each is related to either god's willingness or magic and religion. Very few types of diseases are related to biological reasons. He concluded that the whole system of treatment is related to an established setup of social norms and rituals.

Elwin V., studied the disease and sickness behavior of many tribes. In 1942 (Maria and Suicide), 1942 (The Agaria) 1947 (The Muria and their Ghotul), 1950 (Bondo High Landers) 1954 (The Religions of an Indian tribe) and 1955 (The role of Shamans among the Hill Saora of Orissa). He found that health disease and treatment in these tribes is closely related to their cultural system. He described that there are so many legends and sayings related to different diseases and each disease is related to a particular 'god'. He studied the role of 'Shamans' in treatment of sickness and other problems among Saora Tribe. He wrote "To sick and lonely the 'Shaman' is the nurse and friend and guide, the analyst .... an angel of strength and consolation". Elwin (1955)

Marriott, (1955) studied the health behavior of a Northern Indian Village and he emphasized the cultural definition of medical roles. He opined that trust, responsibility, charity, power, respect - are the important aspects of interpersonal relations in the medical sphere. He found that it is not so much his technical skill that gives prestige to a healer but his spiritual power gained through communion with supernatural entities.

Dandekar and Kumudni (1957), made a demographic survey of six rural communities and found that with a total population of 37,000, there were 730 ailing females and 513 ailing males in the age-group below 15 years and the percentage of getting medical treatment was higher in males than females.

Koos, Es, (1958) Studied the Knowledge and Utilization of Health success by Public Assistance Recipient, and found that the studies from development and developing countries have shown a definite link between low status of women and deficiencies in the knowledge and Utilization of preventive Health services.

Opler (1963) in his study, "the Cultural Definition of Illness in Village India", has listed the following as the most commonly believed causes of various diseases such as Doshas, faulty diet, lack of harmony with the supernatural world, activities of ghosts and witches, displeasure of deities etc.

Khare, (1963) also observed that "The zone of the causative agents of various diseases widens and usually moves towards the supernatural during the period of illness among North Indian Villagers."

Vaidyanathan, KE, (1972) Studied the 'Mortality in India' and found that female mortality in fact is higher for all the three age group, namely, during infancy, childhood and during the productive age, particularly in rural areas, which is the result of neglect of female health.

One most important study of "Primary Health Centres on the Functional Analysis of Health Needs and Science" was done by the Narangwal group at Ludhiana under the auspices of the Johns Hopkins University School of Hygiene and Public Health (U.S.A.) 1972, where attempts have been made to relate health services to the community health needs.

Bhatia (1972), carried out a study on the attitudes of indigenous medicine practioners towards the mulipurpose health schemes.

L.P. Vidhyarthi, (1974) has studied the inter-relationship between Health, Education, Employment and Industry in tribal India and showed the concern with the future of tribes.

Banerjee, (1974) studied health behaviour of rural people in 7 states covering sixteen villages. He observed that most of the villagers, irrespective of their social, economic and occupational status, prefer allopathic medicine. According to Demiguel (1979), "A health system is a set of relationships among institutions, social groups and individuals, that is directed towards maintaining and improving the health status of a population."

Djurfeldt, (1980) emphasized that health is to be seen not merely in terms of curing disease but as an indicator of the level of social, economic, material and environmental development of the country.

Yesudian, (1981) studied the health behaviour of four social classes –high, middle, low and very low-in utilization of health services in Bombay city. He found that as the low and very low social class households are uneducated, their desire to seek health service are also found to be lower than that of middle and high class households. The low class people prefer government hospital and search the place where treatment is offered free of cost.

Srinivasan, (1987) reviewed the efforts of the Government agencies in the delivery of health care services to the rural population since the beginning of the planned era. He found that the people living in interior and remote rural areas, did not have access to the primary health care. The rural health care services suffered from variety of limitations such as insufficiency of medical and para-medical staff, lack of proper accommodation for housing Primary Health Centres, unsatisfactory supply of medicines and equipments and their maintenance etc.

Another study "Women, Family Health and Folk Medicine" (1989) by C. Sridevi, is very much relevant for our study which highlighted the fact that dual system of professional medicine is prevalent in China and South Asia that is the institution of modern medicine exists side by side with folk medical practices. She emphasized that in India, it is more true, specially in case of women and children in rural and tribal areas, which needs the scientific evaluation and authenticity of the system.

Another study "Women's Health and Role in Population Education" (1989) by S.A. Samuel, is also a valuable document which emphasized that women's health issue should not be studied by focussing in health sector alone but it must be dealt along with nutrition programmes, family planning, education, status and employment opportunities, which are related to women's health to a great extant.

'Women's Health' by Gopa Kothari, (1989) deals with the issues like low health status of mothers, maternal morbidity and mortality, mal-nutrition, illiteracy. She came to the conclusion that these are serious matters regarding women's health status which should be removed by the effective measures taken by the Government or relevant agencies.

Developing Women and Children in India (1990) : Edited by Ashok Kumar, is a book which is the collection of many vital researches on issues related to the development of women and children including nutrition and health. The book emphasizes the fact that women and children, by their very nature, are an inter-disciplinary area of knowledge and works; so both the subjects should be studied with integrated point of view.

Hema and Murlidharan, (1993) pointed out, how the policy makers failed to perceive family planning issues as part of the larger problems involving gynecological illness, maternal and child health, sexually transmitted diseases, abortion rights and women's own perspectives and choices.

Vijay Kumar and Chakrapani, (1995) made conclusion that most of the people were not utilizing the services mainly due to the lack of proper transportation facilities and because they were losing faith in Government Health Services due to poor management. Apart from these factors, illiteracy and lack of health consciousness resulted in the most people not being aware of the illness at a stage when prevention is possible.

Studies by (Banerjee, D 1995, Newsletter IX, No. 1, January-February), "Foundation for Research in Community Health" - "Real Threat to Dignified Health Care", New Delhi : (Jay Medical Publication 1992), Banga, Ved Prakash, 1996 "National Health Policy and its Implementation", (Economic and Political weekly, 22 January, pp. 105-08 by Banerjee D. 1995), "Tribal Eco-Health" (C.H. Jill and Geeta Menon, 1994), "A Decade Towards Health for All" (Recommendation of the ICSSR-ICMR panel) "Social Science and Health" (ICSSR, 2.4 Jan-March by Chaterjee, 1993), "Foundation for Research in Community Health" 1989 by Duggal Ravi and Sucheta Amin, are all valuable documents from both points of view i.e. the availability of medical and health care system in the various areas and States of the country and the real condition of people, specially women and children from the health point of view. These studies critically evaluated the present system of Medical and Health Care and reached the conclusion that efforts made by the Government so far, are scarce with the growing needs of increasing health problems.

Qadeer, (1998) suggested that from a public health perspective, two things are clearly needed. First, within reproductive health, priorities should be clearly articulated and reflected in the budgetary allocations. Secondly maternal and child health, nutrition, contraceptive services, and communicable disease control must be integrated within the sphere of the health service system. This will provide a solid foundation for women's health including their reproductive health.

Hygiene, First Aid & Home Nursing (2000) by Usha Mehta & Alka Aggarwal (Hindi Edition)- highlights the adverse effects of child marriage, purdah system and defective methods of family planning on women's health. They emphasized the utility of Primary Health Centres and Maternity Centres for poor class women and children which are inadequate in the country in number and quality.

"Women's Reproductive Health in India" (2000) edited by Radhika Ramasubbam and Shireen J. Jejee Bhoy, provides a comprehensive up-to-date overview of the reproductive and sexual health of women in India. There are ten research articles dealing with various dimensions of the reproductive health situation in India ranging from the situation of adolescents, to the magnitude and patterns of reproductive tract and sexually transmitted infections.

A paper by Shireen J. Jejee Bhoy, titled 'Safe Motherhood in India' is a scholarly research work, which is very much relevant to the present study. The study revealed that maternal morbidity and reproductive morbidity in general, is an outcome of not just biological factors but of women's poverty, powerlessness and lack of control over resources as well. Besides these factors, malnutrition, infection, early and repeated childbearing and high fertility also play an important role in poor maternal health conditions in India. Lack of access to health care along with poor quality of the health delivery system are also responsible factors in this regard.

Another paper, edited in this book "From Contraceptive Target to Informed Choice" by Leela Visaria, is also important in relation to our study. The study emphasized that women should be given autonomy in these matters such as the right to have information about family planning, to decide the number of children, right to control of her body, choice of contraceptives etc.

One more study from above book named "Quality of Care within, the Indian Family Welfare Programme", Gillian Foo and Michael Koenig, unfolds the truth that the medical facilities available in the rural areas are too meagre to serve the purpose of programme. In Government's programme, the key multipurpose extension health worker (ANM) is expected to visit every household within her work area (5,000-6,000 households) at least once in two months to provide family welfare services. The study indicates the significant short comings in worker-client out reach efforts in the frequency and regularity of out reach visits, in the time devoted by workers to outreach activities and in the duration of time spent with clients during outreach visits. There seems poor image and general distrust in the public sector in Health and Family Welfare Programme.

A Scholarly study "Social Policy and Reproductive Health" by Bhanwar Rishysringa, pointed out that reproductive health and rights are not issues that can be solved within the confines of population and health policies. These are fundamentally linked to opportunities for employment and income, control over productive assets and skills and access to public goods and services, in short to create a social situation which put women in command of themselves including their own reproductive health, that means empowerment of women. The study emphasized that for the successful empowerment of women, men too, have to adopt responsible behaviour relating to fertility, disease transmission and child care. Information, education, service back-up and advocacy are also important in the matter of health care.

Om Prakash Sharma, (2000) has examined expansion of the modern health care system and the growing needs of the people because of the rapid pace of population. He observed that poverty squatter and disease go together. Poverty becomes the root cause of mal-nutrition, disease and death. He concluded that progress in medical sciences has increased the life-span of the individual, but due to high cost of modern medical facilities, the poorer sections of society can not take advantage of the system. The health-care delivery system of the government is not sufficient to meet the needs of the down-trodden and vulnerable sections of society in India. He observed that health status is a matter of economic power, so the poorer section of the population suffers badly in maintenance of health and treatment of disease.

Satish Balram Agnihotri (2000), in his scholarly work "Sex Ratio Patterns in the Indian Population", has shed the light on new and challenging aspects of continuous declining proportion of women in Indian population. He discovered that the source of women's oppression does not lie only in poverty, illiteracy, mal-nutrition and the like, but also in prosperity. The findings of the study are based on interdisciplinary approach of economics, demography, development studies and cultural studies. The study is so rational and penetrating that the chairperson of CWDS - Vina Mazumdar has expressed appreciation in the forward of the book in these words "The expanding black regions in Agnihotri's maps ought to convince any one with an open mind that female foeticide and female infanticide are two faces of the same phenomenon where tradition and modernity are not in opposition but in strong alliance." These words are the spoken examples of negation of the health of women even in properous and modern households as well as in poor families.

Venkatesh Srinivasan, (2001) in his recent study "Health and Family Welfare Programme in Developing Countries" has traced the health and family welfare system in India. The author has undertaken the detailed study of innovative activities in the health system of four Indian states with a special emphasis on Rajasthan. He analyzed the three innovations, the first innovation relates to a scheme designed for the girl child, the second relating to the initiation of a large scale community based contraceptive programme and the third is an organizational innovation of starting a communication bureau to consolidate and invigorate the communication activities being undertaken by the health system. In the last chapter of the book, the author proposed a theory for the initiation and implementation of innovations in public system which is very much useful for policy makers, management experts and other scholars who are interested in studying the health and family welfare systems.

N.G.O's as Prime Movers (2001) by : Shivani Dharmrajan, is a book which deals with role of N.G.O's in various sectors of social development, specially with issues like poverty, education, health care, environmental protection and human rights. The Study revealed that Governmental efforts are insufficient in these sectors so the role & responsibility are taken by voluntary organizations.

V. Sujatha, (2003) in her latest study, "Health by the People - Sociology of Medical Lore" has presented the dialectics of the anatomy and interdependence of medical lore in the network of indigenous medical knowledge. The study is based on the field data from Tamil Nadu. The research found that the village folk's medical conceptions and health practices are coherent and live, and make 'health by the people' operational under lived conditions.

'Shakti'-'Multidisciplinary Perspective on Women's Empowerment' in India by Ranjana Harish and Bharti Harishankar, (2003) presents some papers on specific topics relating to women perspective from fine arts, literature, law to social sciences and education. One of the papers titled

'Recognizing Women as Human Resource in Development - A True Way to their Empowerment' is specially relevant to this study. The paper revealed that woman is accepted as National Economic Resource and so her health is of paramount interest for national development.

Critical Evaluation of Review of Literature

As, is apparent from the preceding detailed discussion of existing literature in the field of medical and health sociology in India, specially regarding women's health, attempts made so far, suffer from the following significant limitations.

First - All the studies have a predominant bias being macro studies. Such studies although are useful for understanding the over-all general condition and trends of the problem, but such studies, by their nature, do not touch the core of reality. The correct approach necessarily should be to dissect the problem into small segments and then an intensive effort to assess the reality. The researcher's aim is not to suggest that macro-level studies are useless. What is intended, is to highlight the fact that it is always better to have several micro-level studies before undertaking a macro-level study for making safe generalization at the national or wider social context.

Second, in the present stage of development process in India, rapid changes are taking place, which bring in their trail far reaching changes in socio-cultural and economic-political aspects of life. Therefore, even if a number of micro studies are available in the field, but some new studies in the new areas would have undiluted importance as such as new attempts always are found to throw light on several new facts. In any empirical exercise having a bearing on policy issues, thus, on its own, the necessity of a new micro study remains evergreen.

Third, the fact remains, that none of these studies have taken interest in researching women's health problems in the hilly areas of Uttaranchal Pradesh. The reason may be, that it is a newborn state, which came into existence only in November, 2000. Previously it was a part of a huge state - Uttar Pradesh and was neglected because of its Hilly and Complicated Geographical conditions. So it may fairly be hypothesized that this area of study is unexplored, untraversed and uninvestigated; so the present endeavour is an humble effort to go deep into the ground reality regarding medical and health care of women living in hilly areas of Uttaranchal Pradesh.

The Present Study

The problem under taken in this project, is to study the status and condition of tribal and rural women of hilly areas of Uttaranchal Pradesh, who are the deprived classes of the society. The project is concentrated mainly on the socio-economic profile of the women, their social status and role in the family, their health condition, the attitude of women towards their own health care, specifically towards their reproductive health. At the same time it has thrust upon the study of public health care system, health facilities available in the area, the attitude of women to take benefit of health facilities available in the area, the attitude of male and female members of the family towards the health care of women in the household and finally the role of NGO's, if any, in generating health consciousness among women and efforts made by these NGOs regarding health measures in this region.

The Relevance of the Study

The present study is targeted to health problem of rural and tribal women living in hilly areas of Uttaranchal Pradesh for the following reasons:-

First - Many rural and tribal communities are living in isolated or semi-isolated areas of hills and forests where modern facilities of medical and health care are not available or partially available. So it is the matter of concern to know how they face the situation at the time of health crises;

Second - The health matter, in remote hilly areas of rural and particularly in tribal groups, is, as such a function of the interaction between socio-cultural and socio-biological practices, food habits and nutritional status, the genetic attributes and the environmental conditions, use of herbal drugs, taboos and superstitions which make the health system very much complicated in that areas, which should be studied from socio-analytical point of view;

Third - The hilly region of Garhwal is inhibited by a tribe (Khasa) of Jaunsar Bawar Region, known for its typical family and marriage custom 'Polyandry' which has direct and indirect effects on women's health and demographic balance;

Fourth - Women are the backbone of domestic life, main agency of socialization of new generations. At the same time, women are major part of labour force in the rural and tribal areas of Uttaranchal Pradesh. So their health status must be evaluated;

Fifth - And finally at the last but not the least that health issue of women has multifarious repercussions on the personality and status of women and also on the various aspects of nation's life.

Keeping all the above facts in view, the researcher has decided to investigate the phenomenon of 'Women's Health Status' in hilly areas of Uttaranchal Pradesh.

Objectives of the study

For the present research work **(Medical and Health Care of Women – A Sociological Analysis of Hilly Ares of Uttaranchal Pradesh)** the following objectives have been undertaken -

(i) To assess the socio-economic status of women in hilly areas of Uttaranchal Pradesh;

(ii) To identify the indicators of women's health status;

(iii) To identify the reproductive behavior and attitude towards general health care of women;

(iv) To investigate cultural practices associated with women's medical and health care and its treatment;

(v) To identify the present health care delivery system in hilly regions of Uttaranchal Pradesh by the Government and by the private practitioners or NGO's regarding medical and health care;

(vi) To assess the impact of the National Health Policy and availability of medical health care facilities;

(vii) To identify the pattern of social relationships and the social support system in the villages of hilly areas of Uttaranchal Pradesh.

Formulation of Hypothesis

In a survey type of research work, formulation of hypothesis is not a must step to be undertaken. However to guide the on going exercise the researcher formulated the same in the following terms -

1. Health seeking behavior is culture specific, hence it differs from culture to culture;

2. In tradition bound society the people tend to ignore modern health services available to them;

3. Health status is related to the financial condition of the family : i.e. better economic status would imply better women's health care;

4. Education plays an important role in health seeking behavior of an individual, i.e., educated women are more health conscious than their uneducated counterparts.

Part III

Conceptual Framework

Various concepts are used in this study. These have been briefly explained in the following paragraphs.

Medical Care

The term medical care denotes the "Science or Practice of the Diagnosis, Treatment and Prevention of Disease." (Oxford Dictionary). As a profession, medical care means the service rendered by a doctor or physician to develop better system of healthcare for the people in society.

Traditionally, it was considered as a noble profession. A 'Doctor' or a 'Vaidya' was treated as 'Dhanvantri' (The life giver) and was revered next to God by the patients and their relatives. The spirit of service and altruism were prominent than the value of money or wealth. But now it has become a commercial industry with high profit motive.

Health

Generally, health implies a state of sound and fit body with sound mind, which is able to adapt with the physical environment. But from sociological point of view, health does not mean simply a disease free state of the body, but it is a social phenomenon. As stated by World Health Organization (WHO) "Health is a state of complete physical, mental and social well being and not merely the absence of disease and infirmity." (Preamble to constitution of WHO)

Healthcare includes not only medical care, but also services for promotion of health, prevention of disease, early diagnosis and rehabilitation.

Woman

"The female sex in the species of human race" (oxford Dictionary). Women are generally known to be contextually identified in India as being a daughter, wife and mother. Ensyclopaedia Britanica put the concept in this manner "The very word woman sums up a long history of dependence and subordination." The great historian Gibbon stated that according to ancient law, the woman - a sex created to please and to obey was never supposed to have attained the age of reason. (Kidwai 1978).

According to the constitution of India "women - a weaker section of society - deserving special protection, care and welfare."

Now, after the declaration of women's development decade by the U.N.O., by and large, women are theoretically called as the co-partners in the development process of every country.

Status and Role

Every society is a network of statuses and respective roles. Sociologists and Anthropologists defined 'status' - "The place in a particular system which a certain individual occupies at a particular time, will be referred to as his status with respect to that system". (Linton)

Elliott and Merrill stated that "Status is the position which an individual occupies in the group by virtue of his sex, age, family, occupation, marriage and achievement".

Role and status are the two faces of the same coin. According to Elliott and Merrill "Role is the part which an individual plays as a result of each status." In sociological literature woman's status is often used as a synonym for 'role'. According to Majumdar and Madan "actual treatment, legal status, opportunity for social participation and the character and extent of work, all determine each as a specific sense and manner, the status of women in a society." C.S.W.I.'s view on the status of women is based on the basis of country-wide survey. It opined that "Any attempt to assess the status of women in a society should ideally start from the social-frame-work. Social structure, cultural norms, and value system are important determinants of women's roles and their position in society. The status of any given section of population in a society is intimately connected with its economic position also, which depends on rights, roles and opportunities for participation in economic activities."

In woman's case her status and role in society is determined by social and conventional expectations than her role in economic participation.

Public Health Care Delivery System

Health care delivery system denotes the health care services provided by the government agencies free of cost. It includes not only medical curative measures but also services for promotion of health, prevention of diseases and epidemics and other measures taken in the sphere of hygiene, sanitation and to reduce pollution and other ecological problems.

N.G.Os.

The phrase N.G.O. has been very much in vogue soon after the U.N.O used the term in its documents to mention the Non Governmental Organizations. Previously these types of organizations were called voluntary agencies which seems to be more familiar and have a positive connotation. By its earlier and original meaning "A voluntary organization was a grouping of volunteers joined together with shared value of concerned for a specific goal. The main purpose was to render welfare service to the needy and depressed people." This has been selfless and unpaid service to humanity. But this type of welfare activities is now a gone history.

Today, voluntary organizations consist of full-time paid trained staff of social workers as well as committed professionals from many fields who believe in the specific 'cause' to which they devote their time as a full time activity. (Desai A.S. 1998) In the present scenario N.G.O.s are financially aided by the

Government and they play the bridging role between the people and the Government and they make better rapport with the people.

2

Research Design

Introduction

The quest for novelty is eternal in man. The mysteries of cosmic phenomena have been the fascinating matter of man's curiosity from time immemorial. Being a rational animal, man has been trying to discover and rediscover the complex natural and human phenomena and motivated to enrich his treasure of knowledge through thinking and reasoning day by day, ages by ages. The achievements of material prosperity, culture and civilization of today, is the outcome of man's urge to unfurl the layers of universe and use them for the progress and betterment of humankind. In the process of exploring and understanding, he has tried to know the causal-relations among the various events-natural or human, and draw the conclusions to reach the realm of truth and reality.

Through this 'Gate-way' of reasoning, the man has passed the theological and metaphysical stages of social development and finally reached at the present stage of science and technology-the stage which was named as 'Positive Stage' by August Comte- the father of sociology. With this positive stage of intellectual and rational understanding, the man has tried to uncover the all mysteries of whole universe- the earth, the sky, the sea and human. The scholars of natural and social- sciences called this process of learning, exploring and understanding the truth and reality- 'The Scientific Method.'

Every research work, whether natural or human, has to follow this path of scientific method to reach upto intense-depth to find-out the truth underlying the events. Present study 'The Medical and Health-Care of Women in the Hilly and Tribal Regions of Uttaranchal Pradesh' in the form of major project research work, has also tried to follow the scientific method, tools and techniques and tried to its best to maintain the objectivity in the whole process.

The objectives of any Research may be different and accordingly different designs are planned and executed. Some of the researches may present a true picture of the social problems. While some other researches may aim at finding out the causes of a specific problem, so that a solution may be searched. So the research designs fall into different categories as Exploratory or Formulative design is used to go deep into the causes of some social event or problem - Then there is the descriptive design, which is mainly aimed at finding out the facts and prepare a descriptive report on the basis of those facts. This type of study is based upon scientific tools like interview, observation, questionnaires etc. Another Experimental Research, as Chapin has described it, "The aim of this research is to observe human relationships under certain controlled conditions and situations" just as we do in physical sciences. "Some variables of the problems are controlled and the effect of specific events on the uncontrolled varieties are seen" The Action Research Design is an extended form of the experimental design. Sociologists like Stephen M. Cori have tried to give a specific and concrete form to this design. As Goode & Hatt have put it "The aim of this design is to see change in the present condition whether it is the slum condition, racial prejudice or the efficiency of an organization." Evaluative design, as the name suggests, aims to find the effect or impact of certain programme on the development of a society. Again the pure Research Designs are meant only for the enhancement of knowledge.

Whatever the design of the research may be, the ultimate goal of research is to find out the Truth underlying the events.

As mentioned above that the purpose of the present study is to explore and evaluate the health status of rural and tribal women of Uttaranchal Pradesh, the researcher found necessary and relevant seven objectives, which have been discussed in Chapter I. (See Page no. 45-46, Chapter I)

Area of the Study (Universe)

The researcher has taken the two districts of Uttaranchal State as the Universe of Study because after reviewing the literature, it came to be notice that none of these studies had taken interest in finding out women's health problems in Hilly areas of Uttaranchal Pradesh. The reason may be that it is a new born state which came into existence only in Nov 2000. Previously it was a part of huge state Uttar Pradesh and was neglected because of its hilly and complicated geographical conditions. Uttaranchal is one of the youngest states of India's Republic which came into being on the 9th November 2000 by combining nine northern mountainous districts of Uttar Pradesh viz Uttarkashi, Chamoli, Tehri Garhwal, Dehradun, Pauri Garhwal, Pithoragarh, Almora, Nainital and Haridwar. These nine districts were reorganized into 13 districts.

These are Dehradun, Uttarkashi, Chamoli, Rudra Prayag, Dwarahat, Tehri Garhwal, Pauri Garhwal, Pithoragarh, Champavat, Almora, Bageshwer, Nainital, Udham Singh Nagar. This research is directed to two districts namely Dehradun and Almora.

Salient Features of the Universe

Uttaranchal has been supposed to be the abode of all gods and goddesses. Geographically defined, with the Jammu on West and Tipsy on the east, it includes the sovereign Kingdom of Nepal with the Kali River

The total area of the state of Uttaranchal Pradesh is 53483 sq. km. with a total population of 8479562 lakhs. The ratio of men and women is 1000 : 964. The level of literacy in the state is 72.28% where 60.28% women are literate. This beautiful state, called the abode of gods and Rishis, has a vast and rich culture. For the sample of the present study, out of 13 districts-two districts Dehradun and Almora have been selected purposely. Dehradun from Garhwal region and Almora from Kumaon.

Garhwal means the land of forts. The vast geographical diversity confined with a few kilometers between Tarai and the Himalyan crest has made this land of silvery mountain ranges. From Garhwal Region, Dehradun District has been selected purposely.

Dehradun, the capital of Uttaranchal Pradesh, has been the centre of cultural activity and change, since long. According to Skand Puran, Duv formed part of the region called Kedar Khand. It was included in the Kingdom of Ashoka by the end of 3rd century B.C. For centuries, this region formed part of Garliole Kingdom with some interruption from Rohila. For about two decades till 1815, it was under the occupation of Gorkhas. In April 1815, Gorkhas were ousted from Garhwal and it was annexed by the British. In that year, the region of Dehradun & Jaunsar Bawar were placed under charge of Separate Deputy Commissioner and since 1871, it is being administered as a separate district. In 1965, the district was taken from Meerut division and included in the Garhwal Division.

Dehradun can be divided into two distinct tracts, Mountainous Tract and Sub Mountain tract. The Mountain Tract covers whole of Chakrata Tehsil of the district and consist entirely of a succession of mountains and gorges and comprises Jaunsar Bawar. It is mainly inhabited by the 'Khasa' tribe.

Below the mountain tract, follows the sub mountain, which is the famous Doon Valley bounded by Shivalik Hills in the south and outer scarp of the Himalayas in the North.

Dehradun is chiefly surrounded by dense forests, so forest products play an important role in the economy of the people. It comprised 1477 sq. km. area of Doon.

It has a total population of 12,79,083 lakh. Rural population comprise of 31.44 male 31.66 females, scheduled tribes forming 2.56 lakhs. Dehradun district has been divided into 4 tehsils- Chakrata, Vikas Nagar, Dehrakhas, Rishikesh. Each Tehsil is further divided into Blocks- Chakrata has 2 Blocks- Kalasi and Chakrata. Vikas Nagar is also divided into 2 Blocks namely Sahaspur and Vikas Nagar, Dehra Khas has 3 Blocks namely Raipur, Dehradun and Doiwala. The hilly region of Rishikesh has 2 Blocks namely Doiwala and Rishikesh. Each Block comprises of nearly 50 villages.

The health facilities provided by the government in Dehradun district are – Community Health Centres 4, Primary Health Centres are 22, Maternity Centres are 139.

Kumaon, this name is believed to have been derived from KURMANCHAL meaning the land of Kurmavtar the Tortoi- the incarnate of Lord Vishu, the preserver of Hindu Trinity. Extending from the Northern range of Ganga, plains right upto Tibet, Kumaon's endless panorama of scenic wonders is nothing short of a Romance with pristine and soul lifting nature itself. The Katuri and Chand dynasties glorified the region by constructing some fine temples- now renowned throughout the country. Though largely a Shivalic region, the presiding deity Nanda Devi is among the most exalted deity in Kumaon. From the Kumaon region, the researcher has selected Almora district purposely.

Almora Perched on a hillock at elevation of 1646 m, Almora appears like a large horse shoe. It was in the 16th century capital of Chand rulers. It was under possession of King Kalyuri Baichaldev donated major part of this land to a Gaytre Brahmin Shri Chand Tiwari. Later on when Chand Kingdom was founded in Bora Mandal at the town of Almora was founded centrally located place in 1560M kalian Chand. Almora has an area of 5385 sq km with a population of 630466.

Almora has 3 Tehsils and 11 Developments Blocks, The Tehsils are- Almora, Ranikhet and Bhikia Sein. The Blocks are – Takula, Dhaula Devi, Bhainsa Chana, Lawagara, Hawalbagh, Chaukhutia, Tari Khet, Dwarahat, Bhikia Sain, Sialdey and Sutt. Each block comprises nearly 30 to 50 villages.

The health facilities provided by the government are Community Health Centres-3, Primary Health Centres-8 and Maternity Health Centres are 19.

Reasons for purposive selection of Dehradun District (Jaunsar Bawar Area) & Almora (Kumoun Region)

The study of Jaunsar Bawar is of special interest to the sociologists, because it is inhabited by the Khasra Tribe who have followed different Religio-Social system and remained committed to the theocratic form of Socio-Administrative set up and animistic propitiation in their religious disposition. These tribes, despite modern and social changes, remained regulated by theocratic institutions and animistic cults which have thrived on the practice of appeasement of the deities who have mainly been of malevolent nature, by propitiation rather than worship.

The Khasa are the people of Jaunsar Bawar in the Cis-Himalayan tract. Among them, brothers have traditionally share a wife or wives. Land remains undivided. Wife is taken care by some brothers even if others have to be away. They belong to various Hindu high castes but have been accorded the status of scheduled tribes for the sake of maintaining the legality of polyandry, which is forbidden under Hindu Personal Law. For the sake of special privileges granted to scheduled tribes, these people have developed a stake in the custom and, inspite of changes such as a decrease in its practice and strengthening of the norm of monogamy, like to emphasize its presence. (Quoted from Leela Dube 2001).

The research hypothesized that this custom might have influenced the health and fertility of the women in this area.

This area is also known for secret magical practices under which a widow or infertile woman develops a mysterious power of causing harm to a person just by her so wishing. This is revealed only to her most beloved successor so as to keep this diabolic practice alive. It is supposed to bring prosperity to the community. However, the younger school going girls do not believe in such beliefs and they also did not like the custom of polyandry.

Researcher has selected **Almora** district because of its remoteness, poverty, backwardness and lack of modern facilities.

The project director had done an informal survey of the area under study before taking up the final project. She visited Jaunsar Bawar (Dehraun) with her friend who is teacher in a Jaunsari Village (Kunna Dakura). She got an insight into their culture, way of life and traditions and superstitions and modern impact on their lives. She also visited in some remote villages of Almora with her two friends who are very dedicated social workers of that area and she observed the Kumouni culture and also their problems and miseries.

Sampling Frame

The whole process of sampling, which is adopted for the present study is- Purposive, Stratified and Random depending upon the nature of objectives of the study.

In the initial stage, out of 13 districts of Uttaranchal Praesh, 2 Districts- Dehradun and Almora were selected purposely as mentioned above specifically in the heading 'Area of the Study'. On the next stage, 2 Tehsils from each District – Chakrata and Dera Khas from Dehradun District and Dwarahat and Almora from Almora District were selected purposely too. The purpose was also explained in the above headings. Again 2 Blocks- one from each Tehsil, were selected. At the last stage of sampling process, the selection of villages and households was on random basis. The final sample for the study was of total 600 respondents from various households – 400 from Dehradun and 200 from Almora on random basis according to the size of area and population. Theoretically the total number of respondents constitute the universe of the study. There was some deviation from original sample. Instead of 300 household the researcher selected 400 households from Dehradun District depending upon the demand of the study. Dehradun being larger in area and population than Almora and 200 from Almora District.

Techniques of Data Collection

In this study the following techniques were adopted for data collection -

(i) Interview Schedule

An interview schedule, based on the main objectives of the study was formulated. The topics were divided and subdivided to cover the minutes details related to socio-economic status, medical and health care behaviour, facilities available in the area, socio-cultural beliefs related to the health care and reproductive behaviour etc. interview schedules were pre-tested then finally evolved. Two investigators were appointed for the task- one for Dehradun District another for Almora. Both were qualified and they had proper knowledge of language and remote hilly tracks of their respective areas. Although it was most tedious task due to the need of continuous and strenuous walk over the hills for many meters and kilometers. It took a long time to get the interview schedules filled, going from door to door. The respondents were women of all age groups – the young girls, married young women, old mothers and mothers in law, educated and uneducated. Many times, women were not available due to being busy in either household duties or work out of home such as collecting fuels or fetching water from long distance or work as agricultural labourer etc. Although the task was very much difficult and challenging, but the investigators ultimately won the confidence of respondents and sought their co-operation to large extent.

(ii) Intensive Interview and Observation

To verify the facts and cross check the information supplied by the investigators through interview schedules, and moreover to make the study and research work more reliable, the project director carried out intensive field survey of the area with the help of surpanch, Panchayat members and social workers of the regions under study. She established personal contacts and friendly relations with many young and elderly women and sought interviews and deep information about their health, sanitation, economic condition, work load and attitude of husbands and in-laws towards them in day to day life.

During field-survey and in the process of taking interviews, the project director deeply observed the emotional indicators, physical and mental health condition and financial status of the respondents. This observation proved very much useful to draw the conclusions later.

Some of the primary health centres and one community health centre were also visited by the researcher at the time of their functioning, in both the districts. The information was collected from the doctors, ANMs, menial staff and from patients also to make the Health and Medical Care Scenario more objective and close to reality.

(iii) Collective Interview and Focus Interview

With the help of women panchayat members and social workers, the group interviews were also organized in the local temple campus and at the residence of sarpancha also. In informal chat with fairly large group of respondents, various health issues, such as nutrition, hygiene, problem of water scarcity, family planning, rituals and superstitions related to health of infants and pregnant and lactating mothers were discussed and the women took very much interest in discussion. Some of them were very much excited and keen to tell about the poor health facilities available in their villages. One major issue of prominent discussion was drunkardness of male members of every household which was very much torturous for the health of young married women and the major cause of financial crises in poor households in both the districts.

A few group interviews were taken specially of girl students of class IX and X of some village schools with the permission of school authorities. During interview, the young girls were very much excited, they were inspired to give more and more information about the health behaviour of their family members also. Some class IX, younger girls were shy in nature and they kept quiet all the time during discussion. Some houses were also visited and the actual sanitary and ventilation condition of the residences was noticed. The villages were located too deep so the Project Director had to walk three to four kilometers of steep hills to reach there. Compared to Dehradun, the villages of Almora proved to be very difficult to approach.

(iv) Case Studies

On the basis of individual intensive interviews with some respondents, doctors, ANMs and NGOs, a few case studies have been prepared which are mentioned in appendix 1 in the report.

(v) Additional Aids to Data Collection

To make the study more objective and realistic, the researcher has used camera and tape-recorder.

(vi) Secondary Sources of Data Collection

Although, most of the data has been collected through primary sources mentioned above, but help from secondary data had also been taken. Census Reports, Maps, Journals and Relevant Books from various libraries were also used to make the study more informative.

Processing of Data

After the collecting all 600 interview schedules and completing the intensive field survey, the informations were tabulated mechanically to find out the results.

Interpretation and Analysis

On the basis of data, several tables were designed to find out the information and conclusions. The results were compared across the hypotheses of the study.

Findings and Suggestion

A summary of the whole report and findings were presented. Some suggestions were given which might be used to lessen the health hazards of women living in remote hilly areas.

Limitations of the Study

The study had been concerned with the health problems of women living in remote hilly and tribal villages of Dehradun and Almora Districts, specifically from poor and downtrodden classes. Thus the conclusions drawn from this study may not be applicable to the women from economically well to do households and women, living in Urban Areas of Uttaranchal Pradesh.

It is an academic venture and purely empirical and exploratory sociological analysis, based on the facts obtained through schedules, observation and intensive interviews. The interpretation of facts on the basis of data, had been done, as far as possible objectivity, subject to the constraint of human error.

However, an humble effort had been made to present the true picture of women's health hazards, living in remote Hilly and Tribal Areas of Uattranchal Pradesh, with the hope that the analysis and findings may be used for making proper health policies and programmes to elevate the Health Status of Women.

3

Socio-Economic Profile of the Respondents

Introduction

Socio-Economic Profile provides the base for any sociological enquiry of groups, classes or communities of the People. The identity of a person is recognized through his or her status and role in the system of social structure. An individual member of society is not mere a biological being, but a social being occupying several statuses and roles in society, as observed by Radcliffe Brown (1950). "The components or units of social structure are persons and a person is human being considered not as an organism but as occupying position in a social structure." Eminent social thinker Talcott Parsons (1951) also stated "Social structure is the particular arrangement of the inter-related institutions, agencies and social patterns, as well as social statuses and roles which each person assumes in the group." In his theory of 'Social action' and 'social system' Parsons established that an individual, as a member of society, is not free to act according to his independent will but he has to act in a set of socially patterned behaviour of the socio-cultural system of that society, group or community.

At the same time the status of a person in social hierarchy is decided by his or her age, sex, caste, economic condition, his earning capacity, and his occupational level too. Thus a person's social status, in a given society, is the combined outcome of his position in social hierarchy and his economic achievement.

As far as the question of medical and health care is concerned the studies by Durkheim (1912) Sorokin (1927), Sinha (1951), Ghurye (1961), Dass (1968), Rai (1985), Redcliffe Brown (1971), Muralidharan (1987) revealed that the socio-cultural and economic background play an important role regarding the health behaviour and treatment of illness and diseases of the people.

For the present study, to assess the health behaviour of rural and tribal women of Uttaranchal Pradesh, the researcher has analyzed the components of socio-economic status such as age, marital status, caste, religion, family pattern, educational level, occupational background, sources of income, etc., of the respondents of sample villages.

Regarding the presentation and analysis of data colected through structured schedules, it will be pertinent to mention here that the figures regarding different variables are shown in various tables in two categories – Garhwal (Dehradun District) and Kumoun (Almora District) to juxtapose picture for a comparative look at a glance of the studied areas, but the analysis of variables is presented, taking the view of gross figures, to present an overall picture of the social status of the women of hilly rural and tribal areas of Uttranchal Pradesh and their health related problems vis a vis to the health-care delivery system of the studied areas.

At the same time, some important variables of the socio-economic status, such as caste-structure, economic and occupational status, educational level etc., which have direct impact on the health status of women and also which are important to examine the hypotheses of the study (mentioned in chapter I), have been explained comparatively during analysis, not only on the basis of data shown in the tables, but also with the help of information collected through personal and collective interviews by the Project Director herself, which may sharp the picture better.

Social background

Age

Age is the key variable in determining an individual's power, prestige, privilege and ranking in social life. Biologically age signifies the physical and mental maturity of an individual. Sociologically age denotes the status of an individual in a group, be that his family, kinship or other larger and organized groups within society.

In the present study eight categories of age groups as 0-7, 8-14, 15-21, 22-28, 29-35, 36-42, 43-49, 49 and above were thought suitable for the purpose to inquire the health relating problems and attitude of rural and tribal women of all ages.

As far as the first category of age-group (0-7) is concerned, the question may arise that such small children may not give relevant information related to the study. The researcher's submission regarding this doubt is that, the purpose of the study was to asses the health awareness and health behaviour of women from early childhood to old age. All the eleven respondents (2 from Dehradun District and 9 from Almora) of this category were at the age of 5-7, which is generally considered the school going age. The children from this age-group were asked only basic questions about health, such as physical cleanliness, food habits, playing hobies etc. Regarding disease and medical care, their mothers had given the information during personal and collective interviews.

Table 1 indicates the age-wise breakup of both the regions (Garhwal and Kumoun).

TABLE 1

Showing the Age of Respondents

S.No.	*Age*	*Garhwal*		*Kumauyon*		*Total*	*%*
		f	*%*	*f*	*%*		
1.	0-7	2	0.5%	9	4.5%	11	1.83%
2.	8-14	15	3.75%	8	4%	23	3.83%
3.	15-21	40	10%	21	10.5%	61	10.17%
4.	22-28	135	33.75%	85	42.5%	220	36.67%
5.	29-35	104	26%	53	26.5%	157	26.17%
6.	36-42	64	16%	9	4.5%	73	12.17%
7.	43-49	20	5%	7	3.5%	27	4.5%
8.	49-Above	20	5%	8	4%	28	4.66%
	Total	400	100%	200	100%	600	100%

In the sample of 600 respondents, only 11 (1.83%) belong to the first category of age group, 23 (3.83%) in the second and 61 (10.17%) in the third, 220 (36.67%) in the fourth age group, 157 (26.17%) in the fifth category, 73 (12.17%) in sixth, 27 (4.5%) in the seventh category and 28 (4.66%) belong to the last age category of 49 years and above.

During intensive interview, it was told by the respondents of both the regions that as far as the age and health-care correlation in the present study is concerned the respondents belonging to age group of 22-28, 29 to 35 and 36 to 42, who were fallen in the categories of young daughters-in-law in the households, the other elder members were negligent towards their illness or general weakness. During minor ailments, fever or pregnancy related disturbances; these young daughters-in-law have to work hard in and out of the households. The most privileged classes in the household regarding health care, are children (boys), mothers-in-law and husbands. Good meals, rest and care during illness and treatment of diseases within the limited and rare economic means are the first right of these members of the household.

Religion

From sociological point of view, Religion is one of the most powerful institution, which regulate and guide the individual's actions as well as the source of unity and solidarity of any group or community.

In the present study, the table 2 shows religion wise breakup of the sample. The amazing feature of this study is that in the whole sample of 600 respondents, all have informed that they belong Hindu Dharma.

TABLE 2

Showing the Religion of Respondents

S.No.	*Religion*	*Garhwal*		*Kumauyon*		*Total*	*%*
		f	*%*	*f*	*%*		
1.	Hindu	400	100%	200	100%	600	100%
2.	Muslim	-	-	-	-	-	-
3.	Christion	-	-	-	-	-	-
4.	Others	-	-	-	-	-	-
	Total	400	100%	200	100%	600	100%

Apart from the sample of 600 respondents, the project director herself sought some intensive interviews from more women. Among these, one Christian family came to contact which was converted from high caste Brahmin 'Joshi'.

As far as the relationship between religion and health and treatment of diseases is concerned, religion plays an important role. K.L. Pokrana (1994) observed that "Culture (beliefs and religious practices) defines the sickness and sick-role, its causes and treatment and perspective of health."

Caste

In India, the status of every person is first decided by his or her caste, than by any other factor. 'Caste' is a system of stratification, which is based on the birth of a person, which decides his status, occupation and economic condition in the social hierarchy of any group or community.

Although caste rigidity is decreasing under the influence of modernization process in India, but still it does persist in rural and tribal communities. In rural societies, the caste as a decisive factor to assign the social and occupational status of the individuals and groups, also regulates the health and treatment behaviour.

In the present study, the caste-wise break up is shown in table 3. In the sample of 600 respondents, 314 (52.33%) belong to high castes (Savarna or general), 258 (43%) belong to scheduled castes and 28 (4.67%) were from scheduled tribes (Jaunsari).

TABLE 3

Showing Caste of Respondents

S.No.	*Caste*	*Garhwal*		*Kumauyon*		*Total*	*%*
		f	*%*	*f*	*%*		
1.	General	130	32.5%	184	92%	314	52.33%
2.	Schedule Cast	242	60.5%	16	8%	258	43%
3.	Schedule Tribe	28	7%	-		28	4.67%
	Total	400	100%	200	100%	600	100%

If we examine the easte stucture comparatively of both the regions, the data clearly show that in Garhwal region, majority of respondents belong to either scheduled caste or scheduled tribe from the sample of 400 respondents, while from the sample of Kumoun Region (200), the respondents are mostly from upper castes (Savarna). The impact of caste-structure can be clearly seen on the educational level, economic opportunities and of course on the health status of respondents of both the communities. The correlation between caste structure and educational level may be assessed through the data given in table 4.

During intensive field survey it was observed that high caste women were more health conscious than scheduled caste. But Jaunsari (Tribal) women were also health conscious, although they had some superstitions related to health matters, especially for pregnancy period and some serious and fatal diseases.

Education

Formal education has been considered the most powerful instrument to bring social change and social progress in modern societies and it plays a vital role in person's career, occupation, marriage-prospects, gaining economic stability, prestige and respect and ultimately in gaining the social status in a group or community.

In the present study, the educational level of the respondents of both the regions, is shown in table 4. In the sample of total 600 respondents, 194 (32.33%) were illiterate, 189 (31.5%) have got education up to primary level, 181 (30.17%) up to middle class, 26 (4.33%) were graduates and 10 (1.67%) were Post graduates.

If we compare the educational level of the respondents region-wise the figures indicate that the percentage of illiterate women is quite high (40%) in Garhwal region than Kumoun (17%). As far as the level of education is concerned, the situation of Kumouni women is better than the women of Garhwal. The data indicate that up to primary level 35% women from Garhwal

TABLE 4

Showing the Educational Level of the Respondents

Sl. No.	*Education*	*Garhwal*		*Kumauyon*		*Total*	*%*
		f	*%*	*f*	*%*		
1	Illiterate	160	40%	34	17%	194	32.33%
2.	Primary	140	35%	49	24.5%	189	31.5%
3.	Middle	76	19%	105	52.5%	181	30.17%
4.	Graduate	18	4.5%	8	4%	26	4.33%
5.	P.Graduate	6	1.5%	4	2%	10	1.67%
	Total	400	100%	200	100%	600	100%

are literate, while the percentage of women from Kumoun upto primary level is 24.5%, upto middle class there seems vast gap in the situation as from Garhwal only 19% women took education upto middle class, while from Kumoun, 52.5% women have taken education upto middle class. Although upto graduation level, the situation of both the regions is almost the same but the number of post graduate women is again higher in Kumoun (2%) than Garhwal (1.5%).

One possible reason of this difference in educational level came into notice when the figures related to caste-structure of both the communities were observed minutely. Table 3 is showing the caste-structure of both the communities. It indicates that in the sample of Garhwal region, only 32.5% respondents were from general category (savarna) caste and 60.5% were from scheduled castes and 7% respondents were from scheduled tribe (Jaunsari). While from the sample of Kumoun region as much as 92% respondents were from general category of caste and most of them were from upper castes. Only 8% respondents were from scheduled castes, none from scheduled tribe.

During informal interview and collective interviews with the scheduled caste respondents, the fact came to light that due to lack of agricultural land, most of the girl children stay at home either to lookafter their younger sisters and brothers, or they do household chores, because their mothers had to go out of home for economic earning. So due to lack of opportunity for education and culturally backwardness, the women of scheduled castes and down trodden, have to remain illiterate. They can not afford to send their daughters, even to village primary 'Pathshala'. Very small number of girls could get education upto primary level among these low castes respondents.

The situation of respondents from sawarna and upper-castes of both the regions, was a bit different, during infromal interview, it was observed that women, from these strata of both the communities, more or less they themselves were educated and despite hard-life and economic hardships, they send their girls and boys both to school. From educational point of view, Kumouni women being culturally reformed, were more anxious about their daughter's education than Garhwali women.

As far as the correlation between education and health is concerned, no doubt education plays an important role in health matters as Vijay Kumar S. and Chakrapani C (1995) observed that "illiteracy and lack of health consciousness resulted in the most people not being aware of illness at a stage when prevention is possible. Yesudien (1981) also found in his study of rural areas that "educationally backward people have less knowledge about diseases, have less awareness of available health facilities and have less desire to seek health services." But it is not revealed in reference of the present study. As far as the sample from Kumoun region is concerned, although majority of respondents were educated and they were aware of health-care measures, but the decisive factor for deprivation of proper health care and treatment was none, but poor economic condition of majority of households couppled with scarcity of water for cleanliness and even for cooking and drinking and scarcity of Govt. Health care facilities. In Garhwal region, the situation was a bit different. Although the majority of respondents were either illitrate or less educated (upto primary level) but they were less deprived in health matters because being the natives of nearly villages of Dehradun District (Capital of Uttranchal) they had better health care facilities at maternity centres and primary health centres and better transportation facilities made possible for their reach to these centres. Besides this factor, the respondents of this region were more beneficiary in health matters than the respondents of Almora District. In the sample of Garhwal region, majority of respondents were either from scheduled castes or from scheduled tribes. Although they were educationally backward and at the same time were poor also. But due to the effective working of several NGOs and Missionary Hospitals in those rural and tribal areas, they get free medical treatment and care which was not available to such extent to the respondents of Almora District.

So it was observed in reference to the present study that neither education nor low caste status play too much role in health matters. The economic factors, Geographical infrastructure and availability of health care facilities in the area (Government or voluntary or NGOs), these are the major factors in determining the health status of the people.

Marital Status

The institution of marriage is the legitimized gateway to the family. From the sociological point of view, marital status is decisive factor in fixing the role and status of woman in society.

The marriage wise break up is shown in the table 5. In the sample of 600 respondents, 481 (80.17%) were married, 77 (12.84%) were unmarried, 9 (1.5%) were divorced, 25 (4.16%) were widows, 2 (0.33%) were remarried and 6 (1%) were polyandrous.

TABLE 5

Showing the Marital Status of the Respondents

S.No.	*Marital Status*	*Garhwal*		*Kumauyon*		*Total*	*%*
		f	*%*	*f*	*%*		
1.	Married	346	86.5%	135	67.5%	481	80.17%
2.	Unmarried	22	5.5%	55	27.5%	77	12.84%
3.	Divorcee	4	1%	5	2.5%	9	1.5%
4.	Widow	20	5%	5	2.5%	25	4.16%
5.	Remarried	2	0.5%	-	-	2	0.33%
6.	Polyandry	6	1.5%	-	-	6	1.00%
	Total	400	100%	200	100%	600	100%

Regarding the marital status, it is noteworthy here, that out of 28 tribal women (Jaunsari), only 6 have admitted that they are polyandrous (have more husbands than one), and 4 have told the researcher during intensive interview that they are remarried (although they were also polyandrous). Rest of them kept secrecy about their custom of polyandry. It is also noteworthy here, that during the informal chat with the younger girls, it was told the researcher that they don't like this old custom to marry with all the brothers in the family and they will protest against this unjust tradition which is the source of exploitation of women. They told that in their turn, they would marry to only one man. Effect of education, awareness and impact of modernity was creeping slowly even in a remote tribal village of Chakrata Hills (Distt. Dehradun). A changing trend in age-old customs and in life-style was seen in school going young generation.

From the health's point of view marriage based relationships vis a vis to other family members such as husband, in-laws and children etc decide and influence the scale for receiving the quality and quantity of health related facilities in the house-hold, such as nutrious food, care and rest during illness, expenditure and duration of treatment etc. in every society, specifically in rural and tribal societies.

In the present study, during focus interview and personal interviews, it was told that husbands, fathers and mothers–in-law, and male children get preferential facilities in health-care matters while daughters-in-law who are the pivots of the whole household, when fallen ill, get least care, rest, nutrition and treatment of illness and diseases. The attitude of in-laws towards their daughters in law is negative and uncompassionate. It was informed by the young women that even during pregnancy period, minor fever, headache, backache, they perform all household chores single-handedly and fetch the water to steep-heights for all purposes such as drinking, bathing and food preparation and so on.

It was also came in light that the widows and oldest women of the household such as great grand mothers, they are the last persons to receive care and treatment during illness, they should be contented with house made herbal medicines, liquids and tea etc.

One more point should be noted here that the concept of remarriage of very young widow was forbidden in Kumouni (Almora Distt.) society and was seemed out of question there, but in Garhwal (Dehradun Distt.) there was some relaxation in this matter and it was told that in very genuine case, remarriage of young widow should be permitted.

Family pattern

Family is the basic unit of society. It is the matrix of socialization. Human personalities are forged and shaped on the basis of familial-cultural moulds. Family organization is the basic core of a given society's sex-based division of labour, marital norms and a system of control over resources, rights, duties and privileges of the members. From the health point of view, the type of family pattern plays an important role, specifically in woman's case. The size of family, the number of children, number of male and female members in the house-hold and the status of women in the family-hierarchy, all these familial factors affect the woman's access to health care, nutrition and treatment of illness and diseases etc.

Out of the six hundred sample 248 (41.33%) respondents belong to nuclear type of family, 292 (48.67%) belong to joint family, only 2 (0.33%) have reported belong to extended family, 4 (0.67%) families were headed by only mothers (with children) and 54 families (9%) were headed by only fathers with children.

In the present study data regarding family types is presented and analyzed as under (Table 6)

TABLE 6

Showing Family Pattern of Respondents

S.No.	Type of Family	Garhwal		Kumauyon		Total	%
		f	%	f	%		
1.	Nuclear Family	160	40%	88	44%	248	41.33%
2.	Joint Family	180	45%	112	56%	292	48.67%
3.	Extended Family	2	0.5%	-	-	2	0.33%
4.	Only Mother & Children	4	1%	-	-	4	0.67%
5.	Only Father & Children	54	13.5%	-	-	54	9%
	Total	400	100%	200	100%	600	100%

Occupational Position

Occupation is a clear indication of social status, prestige and economic capacity of a person or of a household in any group, community or society. Health-care and treatment of illness and diseases are the most essential items in every household, but the quality of health care and the treatment depends on the income of the family.

The data regarding occupational status of the respondents, in the present study, is given in the table 7. Out of 600 respondents, 448 (74.66%) belong to agricultural class – 292 (73%) from Garhwal and 156 (78%) from Kumoun. 24 (4%) – 8 (2%) from Garhwal and 16 (8%) from Kumoun are in business class, but they have some land for growing vegetables and maize for home consumption, 108 (18%) – 96 (24%) from Garhwal and 12 (6%) from Kumoun belong to service class, they also have some land for home consumption crops, 128 (21.33%) – 116 (29%) from Garhwal and 12 (6%) from Kumoun have no land and they belong to labour class, 168 (28%) – 102 (25.5%) from Garhwal and 66 (35%) from Kumoun have some land but their major source of livelihood is cattle breeding and belong to pastoral class 52 (8.66%) – 40 (10%) from Garhwal and 12 (6%) from Kumoun have some land and they also perform other activities to meet the family expenditure.

TABLE 7

Showing the Nature of Occupation of the Respondents

Sl.No.	*Occupation*	*Garhwal*		*Kumoun*		*Total*	*%*
		f	*%*	*f*	*%*		
1.	Agriculture	292	73%	156	78%	448	74.66%
2.	Business	8	2%	16	8%	24	4%
3.	Service	96	24%	12	6%	108	18%
4.	Labour	116	29%	12	6%	128	21.33%
5.	Cattle Breading	102	25.5%	66	33%	168	28%
6.	Others	40	10%	12	6%	52	8.66%
	Total						

To assess the economic status of respondents in general, family's **total income** (agriculture coupled with other sources of income) was also inquired. The results in table 8 show very dismal picture of both the communities i.e. Garhwal and Kumoun. Out of 600 respondents 294 (49%) i.e. 242 (60.5%) from Garhwal and 52 (26%) from Kumoun have told their family income below Rs. 2000/- per month, 169 (28.16%) i.e. 116 (29%) from Garhwal and 53 (26.5%) from Kumoun have told below 5000/- per month, 82 (13.68%) i.e. 28 (7%) from Garhwal and 54 (27%) from Kumoun have told below 8000/- per month and only 55 (9.16%) i.e. 14 (3.5%) from Garhwal and 41 (20.5%) from Kumoun have reported their monthly income above eight thousands.

TABLE 8

Showing Income Level of Respondents

Sl.No.	*Monthly Income (In Rs.)*	*Garhwal*		*Kumoun*		*Total*	*%*
		f	*%*	*f*	*%*		
1.	0-2000	242	60.5%	52	26%	294	49%
2.	2000-5000	116	29%	53	26.5%	169	28.16%
3.	5000-8000	28	7%	54	27%	82	13.68%
4.	8000-Above	14	3.5%	41	20.5%	55	9.16%
	Total	400	100%	200	100%	600	100%

The data regarding occupational position and total income, although, presents a desperating picture of both the regions, but in comparison to Garhwal, the economic status of Kumouni women seemed a little better according to the figures available in tables. But through intensive survey by the project director her self to assess the real picture of the problem, the situtation seemed different. During visit in a village, 7 to 8 kilometers far away from Almora city, in a focus interview with approximately 60 housewives of age group in between 25 to 60 years, it was told by all the women that their families had agricultural land sufficient to meet the needs up to subsistence level, five years ago. But the government of Uttaranchal Pradesh has acquired their land for making Base Hospital near by their village. The government officials gave assurance to them for proper compensation of land and the confirmed employment to one person in every family. Now the hospital is in working process since last two years, but neither they got full compensation, nor employment. Now the male members work as labourers on daily wages and the women of every household are maid servants in houses nearby city in well to do families. They are leading very hard economic life and are morally depressed due to loss of their own land. Same condition was also observed in one more village of Kumoun Region, where majority of families belong to so called low castes (Dalit Castes). They have land but very small (Uneconomic holdings). So both men and women have to work as daily wage labourers, specially women are doing hard work to pull-on the family 's expenses because men of hills are mostly, habitual of drinking cheap wines and other Alcoholic drinks and side by side they kill their whole day in playing cards. The total burden of the household, whether domestic chores or earn money, in the most of hilly regions, is on the shoulders of women. Despite this hard labour, researcher was informed by women that wife battering by drunkard husbands is the fate of every woman of both the regions.

To assess the economic status of the respondents, one more item to inquire was considered appropriate and that was the ownership and condition of **residence**. The data regarding this question is shown in the table 9. During interview, it was informed by the respondents that in those hilly regions every household has its own house whether small or big or Kachha (of mud and straw) or pakka (of stones and bricks). The table indicates that out of 600 respondents, 174 (29%) i.e. 134 (33.5%) from Garhwal and 40 (22%) from Kumoun have Kachha house and 426 (71%) i.e. 266 (66.5%) from Garhwal and 160 (80%) from Kumoun have Pakka house.

TABLE 9

Showing the condition of Residence of the Respondents

Sl.No.	*Residence*	*Garhwal*		*Kumoun*		*Total*	*%*
		f	*%*	*f*	*%*		
1.	Kachha House	134	33.5%	40	20%	174	29%
2.	Pakka House	266	66.5%	160	80%	426	71%
	Total	400	100%	200	100%	600	100%

Regarding the condition of residence, it was told that 98% houses in hills are not bad in terms of ventilation and sunlight. And 95% households have cattle shed in or out of house whether Kachha or Pakka. There is no problem of pollution in village areas as such. Most of the houses (75%) have separate kitchen and approximately 70% have more than two rooms in their houses.

TABLE 9 A

Condition of Residence (Size)

Sl.No.	*No. of Rooms*	*Garhwal*		*Kumoun*		*Total*	*%*
		f	*%*	*f*	*%*		
1.	1-2	188	47%	20	10%	208	34.67%
2.	2-4	196	49%	79	39.5%	275	45.83%
3.	4-Above	16	4%	101	50.5%	117	19.5%
	Total	400	100%	200	100%	600	100%

TABLE 9 B

Light and Ventilation

Sl.No.	*Light and Ventilation*	*Garhwal*		*Kumoun*		*Total*	*%*
		f	*%*	*f*	*%*		
1.	Yes	392	98%	196	98%	588	98%
2.	No	8	2%	4	2%	12	2%
	Total	400	100%	200	100%	600	100%

TABLE 9 C

Separate Kitchen

Sl.No.	*Separate Kitchen*	*Garhwal*		*Kumoun*		*Total*	*%*
		f	*%*	*f*	*%*		
1.	Yes	296	74%	154	77%	450	75%
2.	No	104	26%	46	23%	150	25%
	Total	400	100%	200	100%	600	100%

TABLE 9 D

Cattle Shed

Sl.No.	*Cattle Shed*	*Garhwal*		*Kumoun*		*Total*	*%*
		f	*%*	*f*	*%*		
1.	Yes	374	93.5%	198	99%	572	95.33%
2.	No	26	6.5%	2	1%	28	4.67%
	Total	400	100%	200	100%	600	100%

As far as the health status is concerned, the economy of household has very much effect in this matter. The quality of health-care and treatment depends on the income of the family. Many studies (Desai, 1966, Mathews, 1979, Djur feldt, 1980) reveal that there was a significant relationship between economic well-being and kind of food intake, type of treatment during illness and disease.

But the results available of the present study through collected data and also through personal and collective interviews of both the regions i.e. Garhwal and Kumoun, it was observed that, in these remote hilly regions, the matter of health care is very much complicated and multifactoral phenomenon. Economic status, although plays decisive role in health matters in these regions too, no doubt, but at the same time, plenty of economic means, many times does not work due to long distance, steep hilly and dangerous tracks and scarcity of proper health-care institutions in the villages and scarcity of pure drinking water, the patients of serious condition or pregnant women at the time of complicated delivery cases, many times, have to meet ill fate, despite the enough economic means, due to these circumstances.

4

Health Indicators and Attitude towards General Physical Health of Respondents

Introduction

Conventionally, health has been defined in terms of biologically normal and fit condition of the body and mind. Any disorder in health system is termed as illness or disease. The treatment of illness or disease was generally linked with the conjures of doctors and medical experts, whose major function was to try to restore the sick person to health through treatment of one sort or another. But, during the past half era, there seems a fundamental shift in society's attitude towards health care due to the emergence of medical sociology. Departing from the prior definition of health, which emphasized the absence of disease, a few scholars of medical sociology have felt the need to redefining the concept of health. Henry-E-Siegrist wrote "Health is therefore, not simply the absence of disease : it is something positive....." Siegrist (1941). The same point of view was also stated in the constitution of World Health Organization (WHO, 1947) "Health is a state of complete physical and social 'well-being' and not merely the absence of disease or infirmity." This definition, which specified the term 'social well being' gave the new horizons to the concept of health. Now the Health is seen as a capacity to perform, as a state of being required to pursue specified aspirations and for individual fulfillment and for living fully in social environment. This view provided a new thinking to the doctors and nurses and other medical professionals too. They are now focusing on the 'well' rather than the 'sick' (S. Taylor, 2003). He further observed that "Screening programmes set-out to discover signs of disease before they are presented in the surgery, and people are bombarded with information about what they could, and should be doing to lead healthier lives." Taylor (2003).

With the emergence of this new trend many scholars of health research have criticized the modern medical establishments, which have created a cynic and crazy health care environment with the abandon of supplies of medical drugs and equipments which has created a social 'iatrogenesis', i.e. "sponsoring sickness by creating unrealistic health demands that can then only be met by more health care and greater consumption of medical products..... And are also becoming subject to scrutiny and control of health professionals." (Illich 1990). Illich further argued that, "people should fight back against medical dominance over their lives and should freer to take more responsibility for their health care". As a measure for disease prevention and health promotion, this argument or thesis explained by Illich is very much valuable in modern age of materialistic way of life and is very much near to the popular principle for health that 'prevention is better than cure'. But the critics, such as Szreter (1988), Lefanu (1999) and Bunker J. (2001) have stated that "in enthusiasm to criticize the 'Medicalization', the critics have failed to take into account the contribution of clinical medicine to improving the quality of people's lives by, for example, controlling pain, improving eyesight and restoring mobility and to longevity as well."

No doubt, modern medical system has contributed a lot in reducing the death rates due to epidemics, infant mortality during birth infections and many other fatal diseases. The credit of increasing expectancy of life since last ten decades in India and more in developed countries, also goes to modern clinical system to large extent. But the fact remains beyond doubt, that excessive dominance and monopolistic control of medical professionals and medicine companies over people's lives has a damaging effect on social life, which creates a kind of slavery and over dependence on medicines and drugs. Illich (1990) observed that, "Experiences once seen as a normal part of the human condition, such as pregnancy and child-birth, growth during childhood and adolescence, aging and dying have now been brought under medical jurisdiction." Moreover "there are many stressful events in persons' lives such as bereavement, unemployment, financial crisis, divorce or widowhood etc., these also can make people more vulnerable to illness or premature death." S. Taylor, David Field (2003). These stressful life events produce bio-chemical changes in the body that weaken its immune system and leave the individuals more vulnerable to disease. These situations of human lives are not mere the subject of medical science. "In this context, sociological work has explored the relationship between people's health and their interactive social networks." S. Taylor (2003).

Through this theoretical discussion, the researcher wants to say that in recent years, it has been realized by many scholars, that health depends on less on what doctors and nurses do for patients and more on what people do for themselves. Although the approach is not new because thousands years ago the great Indian seers have prescribed the 'Yogic way' of life to remain healthy and active. This approach is the revival of that old precious formula for health and on the pattern of life, which they lived. This recent approach towards health is termed by social scientists as "behavioural approach". The researchers of this ideology have concluded that, "health and longevity are increased with the number of health rules followed by the people." Mc Keown (1979). At the same time, it is realized that health care network is linked with the fabric of social and cultural setup of a particular society, which decides the behaviour seeking attitude of the people to large extent.

In the present study, to assess the health behaviour of the rural and tribal women of Uttaranchal Pradesh, some important aspects of behaviour, related to health such as personal hygienic, food habits, general condition of physical health, capacity and duration of working hours, attitude and awareness towards their health care, attitude towards reproductive behaviour (for married women) and cleanliness during monthly periods etc. were thought appropriate for inquiry.

Personal Hygiene

Personal hygiene is one of the most important factor which affects the health of an individual primarily. Although personal hygiene is the matter totally concerned with individual's own thinking, habits and practice, but sociologists do not treat it as an absolute individual matter but relative to socio-cultural and economic conditions of a society.

In the present study the women of two hilly regions – Garhwal (Dehradun District) and Kumoun (Almora District) expressed their view in terms of environmental and geographical conditions of the region and not in terms of religious or ritual prevailing. The data collected regarding various essential components of personal hygiene such as bathing, cleaning of teeth, hair, nails, clothes and cleanliness during monthly periods etc. are shown in table 1.1 to 1.6.

Table 1 indicates that out of 600 respondents, 197 (32.83%) take bath every day, 276 (46%) twice in a week and 127 (21.17%) take bath once in a week. Table 1.2 shows that 86 (14.33%) wash hair daily, 301 (50.17%) twice in a week and 213 (35.5%) once in a week. Table 1.3 shows washing of clothes, which was done by 183 (30.5%) daily, 123 (20.5%) twice in a week and 294 (49%) once in a week. Cleanliness of teeth is showing in table 1.4 which indicates that 519 (86.5%) clean daily, 74 (12.33%) twice a day and 7 (1.16%) have reported that they do not clean daily but some times. Table 1.5 shows nail cutting and cleaning, 347 (57.83%) clean daily, 32 (5.33%) twice in a week, 81 (13.5%) once in a week and 140 (23.34%) some times.

TABLE 1.1

Information Related to Take Bath

Sl.No.	*Taking Bath*	*Garhwal*		*Kumoun*		*Total*	*%*
		f	*%*	*f*	*%*		
1.	Daily	184	46%	13	6.5%	197	32.83%
2.	Twice a week	116	29%	160	80%	276	46%
3.	Once a week	100	25%	27	13.5%	127	21.17%
	Total	400	100%	200	100%	600	100%

TABLE 1.2

Information Related to Cleanliness of Hair

Sl.No.	*Cleanliness of Hairs*	*Garhwal*		*Kumoun*		*Total*	*%*
		f	*%*	*f*	*%*		
1.	Daily	52	13%	34	17%	86	14.33%
2.	Twice a week	152	38%	149	74.5%	301	50.17%
3.	Once a week	196	49%	17	8.5%	213	35.5%
	Total	400	100%	200	100%	600	100%

TABLE 1.3

Information Related to Cleanliness of Clothes

Sl.No.	*Cleanliness of Clothes*	*Garhwal*		*Kumoun*		*Total*	*%*
		f	*%*	*f*	*%*		
1.	Daily	160	40%	23	11.5%	183	30.5%
2.	Twice a week	60	15%	63	31.5%	123	20.5%
3.	Once a week	180	45%	114	57%	294	49%
	Total	400	100%	200	100%	600	100%

TABLE 1.4

Information Related to Teeth Cleaning

Sl.No.	*Teeth Cleaning*	*Garhwal*		*Kumoun*		*Total*	*%*
		f	*%*	*f*	*%*		
1.	Daily	324	81%	195	97.5%	519	86.5%
2.	Twice a day	72	18%	2	1%	74	12.33%
3.	Not Daily But Some Times	4	1%	3	1.5%	7	1.16%
	Total	400	100%	200	100%	600	100%

TABLE 1.5

Information Related to Nails Cleaning

Sl.No.	*Nails Cleaning*	*Garhwal*		*Kumoun*		*Total*	*%*
		f	*%*	*f*	*%*		
1.	Daily	342	85.5%	5	2.5%	347	57.83%
2.	Twice a week	16	4%	16	8%	32	5.33%
3.	Once a week	28	7%	53	26.5%	81	13.5%
4.	Some Times	14	3.5%	126	63%	140	23.34%
	Total	400	100%	200	100%	600	100%

One most important aspect from hygienic point of view for young and adult women is to maintain the cleanliness during monthly periods. Table 1.6 shows that out of 600 respondents, the question was applicable to only 544 respondents, 56 were either below age or were above the age of 50 years. Out of 544, 516 (86%) have reported that they use clothes during that period and the same clothes were used repeatedly after washing them. Only 3 (0.5%) have reported the use of cotton and 25 (4.17%) told that they use sanitary napkins.

TABLE 1.6

Information Related to Cleanliness during Monthly Periods

Sl.No.	*Kind of Means*	*Garhwal*		*Kumoun*		*Total*	*%*
		f	*%*	*f*	*%*		
1.	Clothes	368	92%	148	74%	516	86%
2.	Cotton	2	0.5%	1	0.5%	3	0.5%
3.	Sanitary Napkins	18	4.5%	7	3.5%	25	4.17%
4.	Not Applicable	12	3%	44	22%	56	9.33%
	Total	400	100%	200	100%	600	100%

During intensive survey by the researcher of some villages of Almora district and informal discussion with few women in a group, some serious issues were brought to notice, which could not be ignored. The bare reality is that, there are so many environmental and geographical factors linked to peoples health that are out-side the direct control of people's own behaviour, which are hindrances in the practicing of hygienic health measures, for example the poor availability of water in remote hilly area. The women of a surveyed village told that there is a great crisis of even drinking water and water for essential domestic needs such as cooking food and cleaning utensils etc. The question of bathing and washing of clothes, and hair every day is impossible for them. Only a few prosperous households could manage the 'luxury' of taking bath daily. The project director herself has noticed during intensive field survey in the month of mid June in Almora district that nearly 50 to 60 women (mostly from Dalit caste) of a village near by an important tourist point of Almora (Binsar) were waiting for two to three hours for a Tanker of water which was arranged by the village surpanch from district water supply department, because, they told, that the natural sources of water available in the village were badly dried up due to deforestation policy and other ecological imbalances even in that remote and peaceful and secluded hilly regions. So it was observed that although the women of that region were aware of hygienic way of living but the environmental conditions do not allow them in practicing. Besides this, in the months of December, January and February, there is heavy snowfall in many villages, so the water crisis and acute cold weather, both create problems to follow hygienic rules properly. So the concept of personal hygiene, in these hilly regions, is very much relative to their environmental conditions.

Food Habits

Health and food are inseparable aspects of human body and mind. The regularity of circulatory system, the energy of nervous system and the life of cells and strength of muscles and tissues of every organ of the body, depends on the nutritive value of food-stuffs which a person eats every day. The built and growth of a child in mother's womb is the outcome of that diet which a woman takes during her pregnancy period. So it may be said that a person's origin, existence, growth of organism, strength, capacity to work and to bear the environmental crisis – all are related to the kind and quality of food which he or she takes in their daily routine.

In the present study, to inquire the food habits and the quality and variety of food items which are the part and parcel of daily routine of the women of Uttaranchal Pradesh, the three points were thought sufficient in this regard i.e. – vegetarian–non-vegetarian, the variety of food materials and frequency of food intake in a day. These components are indicated in tables 2.1 to 2.3.

TABLE 2.1

Information Related to Frequency of Food Intake

Sl.No.	*Frequency of Food Intake*	*Garhwal*		*Kumoun*		*Total*	*%*
		f	*%*	*f*	*%*		
1.	Once	40	10%	-	-	40	6.66%
2.	Twice	316	79%	68	34%	384	64%
3.	More than two times	44	11%	132	66%	176	29.34%
	Total	400	100%	200	100%	600	100%

Table 2.1 indicates that out of 600 respondents 40 (6.66%) take food only one time in a day because they have to do hard work in the households and out of home as labourer on daily wages. So they could manage to cook proper meals only once in a day in the evening, rest of the day, they somehow kill their appetite with tea and so on. 384 (64%) take proper meals twice

in a day but no breakfast in the morning. 176 (29.34%) take more than two times including breakfast.

Table 2.2 indicates that 249 (41.5%) respondents are only vegetarian and 351 (58.5%) are non-vegetarian, but they take vegetarian food also side by side. As far as the question is of variety of food-stuffs, all vegetarian and non vegetarians told that they take food-grains (rice is more popular than wheat), pulses, vegetables and fruits, because most of the households have their own kitchen gardens and small terraced fields. They grow many eatables in their own fields. They take only those vegetables and grains which are available in their fields. They have no spare money for purchasing other fruits and things from the market. Some of them make exchange in weekly village Hatts, many times they may not get vegetables or fruits due to seasonal factors. Most of the households in hilly regions are under nourished due to poverty and overburden of labour.

TABLE 2.2 A

Information Related to Kind of Food

Sl.No.	*Kind of Food*	*Garhwal*		*Kumoun*		*Total*	*%*
		f	*%*	*f*	*%*		
1.	Vegetarian	208	52%	41	20.5%	249	41.5%
2.	Non-Vegetarian	192	48%	159	79.5%	351	58.5%
	Total	400	100%	200	100%	600	100%

It would be proper to mention here that food habits are also out of control of person's wish or choice or in terms of nutritive values, because to manage the quality of food items depends on the purchasing power of the household and also on the availability of the variety and quality of food items in the particular region.

During field survey, it was observed by the researcher that the life in these hilly regions is economically very hard and most of the people are living on the verge of subsistence level economy there. So the question of taking nutritive food and fruits or other delicious and healthy edibles is not seemed so relevant there. The important problem is to manage food somehow to live alive and to do hard labour.

TABLE 2.2B

Information Related to Variety of Food Items

Sl.No.	*Type of Food*	*Garhwal*		*Kumoun*		*Total*	*%*
		f	*%*	*f*	*%*		
1.	**Vegetarian**						
(A)	Grains	280	70%	197	98.5%	477	79.5%
(B)	Pulses	274	68.5%	185	92.5%	459	76.5%
(C)	Vegetable	308	77%	199	99.5%	507	84.5%
(D)	Fruits	196	49%	115	57.5%	311	51.83%
2.	**Non-**						
(A)	**Vegetarian**	228	57%	166	83%	394	65.66%
(B)	Egg	170	42.5%	130	65%	300	50%
(C)	Meat	130	32.5%	98	49%	228	38%
	Fish						
	Total						

General Condition of Physical Health

General physical health of a person is that dynamic condition of body and mind in which he or she performs his roles properly in day to day life with his all organs in healthy and fit condition. M.S. Yadav (1994) stated that, "physical health denotes the mobility and adjustment of organs according to a person's age and weight." The good physical health needs healthy mind as its pre condition. Person with healthy mind and healthy body can face environmental hazards and may achieve his desired goals of life with all his capacities and abilities.

In the present study, to assess the general physical condition of the women of Uttaranchal Pradesh, three components were realized essential to inquire, i.e. their feeling about their own general health condition, total working hours in a day and minor ailments or serious health problems in day-to-day life. These indicators are shown in tables 3.1 to 3.3.

TABLE 3.1

Feeling about General Health Condition

Sl No.	*Condition of Health*	*Garhwal*		*Kumoun*		*Total*	*%*
		f	*%*	*f*	*%*		
1.	Excellent	34	8.5%	19	9.5%	53	8.83%
2.	Good	298	74.5%	151	75.5%	449	74.83%
3.	Sick and Weak	68	17%	30	15%	98	16.34%
	Total	400	100%	200	100%	600	100%

Table 3.1 indicates that out of 600 respondents 53 (8.83%) have reported that they feel quite healthy and excellent about their health, 449 (74.83%) have told that they feel normally good about their health and 98 (16.34%) felt sick and weak.

Table 3.2 indicates that 137 (22.83%) have told that they work only 1 to 3 hours a day. The respondents of this category were either below the age group of 12 and some of them were school going or they were above the age of sixty and perform the role of grand mothers etc. 344 (57.33%) have reported that they work four to seven hours in a day, 114 (19%) have told that they work more than 7 hours in a day. 5 (0.84%) have reported that neither they work in, nor out of house. They were eldest old women of the household. They only observe the daughters inlaw's routine and tells the stories to great grand children or chatting with the old women of neighborhood.

TABLE 3.2

Information Related to Working Hours of Respondents

Sl.No.	*Working Hours*	*Garhwal*		*Kumoun*		*Total*	*%*
		f	*%*	*f*	*%*		
1.	1-3	72	18%	65	32.5%	137	22.83%
2.	4-7	314	78.5%	30	15%	344	57.33%
3.	7-Above	14	3.5%	100	50%	114	19%
4.	Not Working	-	-	5	2.5%	5	0.84%
	Total	400	100%	200	100%	600	100%

Table 3.3 indicates the various minor and major health problems, which the women of hills have to face in their day to day life. Out of 600, 105 (17.5%) have reported that they are suffering from chronic cough and cold, and 549 (91.5%) have told that they have permanent problem of back and body ache because they have to fetch water twice or thrice every day from steep heights, have to work in the fields or anywhere else as labourer for six to eight hours a day and above all they have to walk on steep heights to valley and valley to heights many times a day for some reason or the other. But they have accepted these health problems as their destiny and a normal part of their lives. 45 (7.5%) have reported the problem of Asthema, 75 (12.5%) told that during monthly periods they face the problems of excessive bleeding and weakness, 170 (28.3%) have told that they feel tiredness and weakness all the time even then they do all the work in and out of home. 26 (4.33%) have

reported eye's problems, 8 (1.33%) had ear problems and one woman was suffering from Cancer, 2 (0.33%) had heart problem and 1 women (0.17%) had some injury.

TABLE 3.3

Information Related to Type of Diseases

Sl.No.	*Type of Diseases*	*Garhwal*		*Kumoun*		*Total*	*%*
		f	*%*	*f*	*%*		
1.	Cough and Cold	86	21.5%	19	9.5%	105	17.5%
2.	Body and Backache	385	96.25%	164	82%	549	91.5%
3.	Breathlessness and Asthma	36	9%	9	4.5%	45	7.5%
4.	Excessive Bleeding	74	18.5%	1	0.5%	75	12.5%
5.	Weakness	144	72%	26	13%	170	28.3%
6.	Heart Problem	-		2	1%	2	0.33%
7.	Eye Problem	24	6%	2	1%	26	4.33%
8.	Ear Problem	6	1.5%	2	1%	8	1.33%
9.	Injury	-		1	0.5%	1	0.17%
10.	Aids	-		-		-	-
11.	Cancer	-		1	0.5%	1	0.17%
	Total						

Attitude towards General Health and Medical Care during Illness

"It is generally agreed that sickness and diseases are universal threat to individual's and group's survival." Coe, RM (1978). Even minor disorder in the body system creates restlessness, dullness and depression in person's day-to-day life and affects his capacity and desire to work. So every society, indigenous or modern has searched the ways to combat sickness and diseases, which are institutionally established. "People react to diseases and sickness according to their social and cultural belief system in which they grow and socialized. The care and treatment adopted by the people during illness and diseases are also the outcome of socio-cultural setup. So it is important to understand the attitude and beliefs, the people hold about health and disease." Coe, RM (1978).

In the study in hand, in order to know the general attitude of the women respondents of Uattaranchal Pradesh, four criteria were seemed relevant to this question – One caring or careless about health, two, precautionary measures taken for health, three, general reaction to disease and steps taken during illness, four, sources of medical facilities. These items are shown in tables 4.1 to 4.4.

As apparent from the table 4.1, that out of 600 respondents 532 (88.67%) have reported that they are careful about their health, only 68 (11.33%) have told that they don't bother minor ailments and are not very much particular about their health.

TABLE 4.1

Attitude towards General Health Care

Sl.No.	*Condition of Health*	*Garhwal*		*Kumoun*		*Total*	*%*
		f	*%*	*f*	*%*		
1.	Caring	348	87%	184	92%	532	88.67%
2.	Careless	52	13%	16	8%	68	11.33%
	Total	400	100%	200	100%	600	100%

Table 4.2 indicates the precaution taken by the respondents in day to day routine such as 524 (87.33%) have told that they wash their hands before cooking the meals and before eating also. 332 (55.33%) have told that they take their meals regular on fixed timings. 241 (40.16%) have reported that they are careful about nutritive value of food as milk, ghee, eggs & meat. 203 (33.83%) take green vegetables and fruits also, 316 (52.66%) have told that although they can't afford these things daily but they take twice or thrice or some times in a week according to budget. As precautionary measures, 381

TABLE 4.2

Precaution taken Regarding General Health

Sl.No.	*Precaution Taken*	*Garhwal*		*Kumoun*		*Total*	*%*
		f	*%*	*f*	*%*		
1.	Washing hands before cooking and Eating	346	86.5%	178	89%	524	87.33%
2.	Fixed times of Meals	194	48.5%	138	69%	332	55.33%
3.	Careful about Nutrition	156	39%	85	42.5%	241	40.16%
4.	In take of green Vegetables and Fruits (Regular)	186	46.5%	17	8.5%	203	33.83%
5.	In take of green Vegetables and Fruits (Some times)	166	41.5%	150	75%	316	52.66%
6.	Rest during Minor Illness or Tiredness	224	56%	157	78.5%	381	63.5%
7.	Overlook the Minor Ailments	136	34%	69	34.5%	205	34.16%
	Total						

(63.5%) have told that during minor illness or fatigue or during monthly periods they take proper rest in between the routine household chores. While 205 (34.16%) women over look fatigue or aching as they could not afford to take rest due to over burden of labour in and out of house.

Table 4.3 indicates the steps taken during sickness and diseases. Out of 600 respondents only 109 (18.17%) have reported that they go to doctor at once for treatment, 98 (16.33%) have told that in primary stage they try home treatment such as herbs, oils, haldi and hot water bottle etc., 82 (13.67%) have told that they go to Hakim Ji or Vaidya for treatment. 38 (6.33%) have told that they perform some religious activities such as Pooja of a particular deity or Havan and Upvas or wearing some sacred thread or Tabeej etc. 219 (36.5%) have told that they do not give much importance to diseases as they come and go when not attended seriously. 54 (9%) have not answered properly and they avoided to talk about this matter.

TABLE 4.3

Step taken during sickness and disease

Sl.No.	*Steps*	*Garhwal*		*Kumoun*		*Total*	*%*
		f	*%*	*f*	*%*		
1.	Going to Doctor	88	22%	21	10.5%	109	18.17%
2.	Home Treatment	96	24%	2	1%	98	16.33%
3.	Hakim or Vaidya	82	20.5%	-	-	82	13.67%
4.	Religious Rituals	36	9%	2	1%	38	6.33%
5.	Over looking Disease	92	23%	127	63.5%	219	36.5%
6.	Not Answered	6	1.5%	48	24%	54	9%
	Total	400	100%	200	100%	600	100%

Table 4.4 indicates the source of treatment. Out of 600 respondents, 342 (57%) have told that they go to government hospitals or dispensaries, because they cannot afford the costly treatment of private doctors, although, government doctors take too much time due to over crowded situation and there is always shortage of costly medicines or injections. 258 (43%) have told that they cannot rely on government agencies due to many inconveniences, so they go to private doctors and nursing homes despite the shortage of finances which they manage anyhow. These respondents were from educated families and they themselves were also educated upto high school and intermediate classes.

TABLE 4.4

Sources of treatment adopted by the Respondents during Illness

Sl.No.	*Sources*	*Garhwal*		*Kumoun*		*Total*	*%*
		f	*%*	*f*	*%*		
1.	Treatment in Government Agencies	290	72.5%	52	26%	342	57%
2.	Private Doctors	110	27.5%	148	74%	258	43%
	Total	400	100%	200	100%	600	100%

5

To Identify the Reproductive Behaviour of the Respondents

The reproductive health of women is the backbone of every family, society and nation. Although reproductive health is the integral part of women's general health, despite the fact, it needs extra care and precautions during specific time and situation.

In modern civil societies, "the reproductive health of women is recognized as a basic human right, without which women can neither, fully play their roles as carers for their families nor as participants in the process of economic and social development." R. Ramasubban, S. J. Jeeje Bhoy (2000). C. F. Brockington (1954) emphasized that reproduction is a normal physical process and women should be healthy in pregnancy period. But the reality of society regarding women's reproductive health is different from this assumption. In under developed and developing countries, the death rate of infants and pregnant women, during pre and post natal periods, was increasing constantly in the first half of the 20th century. To analyze the situation, "The World Health Organization (1948) had enacted a planned policy for the welfare of pregnant mother and child, which was discussed in international seminar on maternal mortality." Markendey Singh Yadava (1994).

In this perspective the U.N. gave a comprehensive meaning to the concept of reproductive health of women "as a state of complete physical, mental and social well being in all matters related to the reproductive system and to its functions and processes". United Nations (1994). According to this perspective, reproductive health encompasses a vast range of health concerns such as : "a satisfying and safe sex life free from the fear of disease; coercion and violence; the capability to reproductive freedom to decide when, and how often to do so; the ability to go safely through pregnancy and child birth and have the best chance of having a healthy infant and the right of access to proper health care services; access to safe and affordable abortion facilities; prevention and care of sexual and reproductive health problems; the right of information of family planning devices etc." Radhika Rama Subban, Shiren J. Jejee Bhoy (2000). All these issues are related not only with bio-medical sphere, but their origins often lie in human behaviour that is embedded in socially and culturally constructed pattern of gender relations. These are in turn, influenced by economic and political factors.

In underdeveloped and developing countries, the rate of mortality and morbidity of pregnant women before and after the birth of child is still very high, due to the negative and narrow attitude of society and the government both, towards the reproductive health of women and due to many other social, cultural and economic factors. In a study 'Safe Motherhood in India' S. J. Jejee Bhoy observed that, "the magnitude of women's reproductive health problems in India is immense. The maternal mortality ratio in India, estimated at 400-570 per 100,000 live births, is fifty times higher than several developed countries and six times higher than neighbouring Sri Lanka. In India, between 4 and 5 million women suffer from ill health associated with child bearing. The reason behind this situation is the prevalence of the narrow conception of women's role in India as connected only with child-bearing while the concept needs to make it a reality. It underlines a commitment to respond to women's health needs throughout their life cycle. It needs to recognize that women's needs are different from men's, both biologically and socially, women's bodies and social realities are different. Women are more disadvantaged than men and their vulnerability to common health risks may be expected to be much greater with additional implications for their reproductive health. The unequal gender relations are also responsible for this situation." R. Ramasubban, S. J. Jejee Bhoy (2000).

Although the majority of maternal deaths and episodes of ill health in India are preventable, but the ignorance and lack of knowledge about sexual behaviour, poverty and socio-cultural framework made the situation worse, specifically in villages and remote tribal areas.

In the present study to assess the reproductive behaviour of the women in hilly and tribal areas of Uttaranchal Pradesh, a comprehensive range of factors, such as attitude towards marriage, number of children, attitude towards family planning measures, precautions taken during pregnancy, medical care during pre and post-natal periods, attitude towards abortion, place and source of child birth, religious or cultural practices (if any) during and after pregnancy, period of rest, special care after child birth, care of infant and so on. These and some other physical, cultural and behavioural factors have been taken into account to make the study relevant and meaningful.

The analysis of the following items with the help of tables will serve the purpose.

The Attitude Towards Marriage and Children

Marriage is considered as an essential social institution to enter in family life and for procreation of new generations, almost in all societies, traditional or modern. In India unlike some other countries, reproduction and fertility of adolescents, young and adults occur mainly within the context of marriage.

In the light of above discussion the data collected for the present study, which is shown in Table 5.1 that out of 600 respondents, 368 (61.33%) women entered into marriage at the age of 15 to 20 years, 149 (24.83%) at the age group of 21 to 25 years and only 6 (1%) were married at the age group of 25 years and above, rest 77 (12.84%) were unmarried.

TABLE 5.1

Information on the Age at the time of Marriage of Respondents

Sl.No.	*Age*	*Garhwal*		*Kumoun*		*Total*	*%*
		f	*%*	*f*	*%*		
1.	15 - 20	238	59.5%	130	65%	368	61.33%
2.	21 - 25	132	33%	17	8.5%	149	24.83%
3.	25 - Above	6	1.5%	-	-	6	1%
4.	Unmarried	24	6%	53	26.5%	77	12.84%
	Total	400	100%	200	100%	600	100%

TABLE 5.2

Information on the Age at First Pregnancy of Respondents

Sl.No.	*Age*	*Garhwal*		*Kumoun*		*Total*	*%*
		f	*%*	*f*	*%*		
1.	15 - 20	136	35.32%	19	13.76%	155	29.64%
2.	21 - 25	175	45.4%	100	72.48%	275	52.58%
3.	25 - Above	24	6.24%	5	3.62%	29	5.54%
4.	Issueless	50	12.99%	14	10.14%	64	12.24%
	Total	385	100%	138	100%	523	100%

The table no. 5.2 indicates the age at first pregnancy. Out of 523 married respondents, 155 (29.64%) have experienced first pregnancy, at the age of 15 to 20, 275 (52.58%) at the age of 21-25 and only 29 (5.54%) have experienced their first pregnancy at the age of 25 years and above. 64 (12.24%) respondents had not experienced pregnancy. They were issueless still.

Regarding the number of children out of 523 married women, 64 (12.24%) were issueless, 321 (61.38%) have reported that they have 1 to 3 children, either sons or daughters or both. 138 (26.38%) told that they have 4 to 6 children, most of them had 2 or 3 daughters as their first, second and third attempt and then they tried one to three times more for a son. The data regarding this information is shown in the table no. 5.3

TABLE 5.3

Information on the Number of Children of Respondents

Sl.No.	*Number of Children*	*Garhwal*		*Kumoun*		*Total*	*%*
		f	*%*	*f*	*%*		
1.	Issueless	43	12.33%	21	12.08%	64	12.24%
2.	1 - 3	214	61.31%	107	61.49%	321	61.38%
3.	4 - 6	92	26.36%	46	26.43%	138	26.38%
	Total	349	100%	174	100%	523	100%

TABLE 5.4

Information on who take Decision Regarding Children from Respondents

Sl.No.	*Who take Decision*	*Garhwal*		*Kumoun*		*Total*	*%*
		f	*%*	*f*	*%*		
1.	Self	6	1.60%	9	6.12%	15	2.87%
2.	Husband	152	40.42%	47	31.98%	199	38.05%
3.	In-Laws	10	2.66%	2	1.36%	12	2.30%
4.	Both	208	55.32%	89	60.54%	297	56.78%
	Total	376	100%	147	100%	523	100%

Table 5.4 indicates the decision taken regarding the number and interval between the children. Only 15 (2.87%) have reported that their consent was primary, 199 (38.05%) told that the decision of husband was only and final, 12 (2.30%) have reported that in-laws have the supremacy in this matter and 297 (56.78%) have reported that husband and wife both take decision in this matter.

Table 5.5 indicates the cases of abortion. Out of 523 married women, 141 (26.97%) had to face abortion, when asked that these were voluntary, forced or natural, they all reported that the abortions were natural. Rest of 318 (60.80%) have told that they went through safe pregnancy and child birth, 64 (12.3%) were issueless.

TABLE 5.5

Information on cases of Abortion of Respondents

Sl.No.	*Abortions*	*Garhwal*		*Kumoun*		*Total*	*%*
		f	*%*	*f*	*%*		
1.	Voluntary	-	-	-	-	-	-
2.	Natural	122	32.45%	19	12.92%	141	26.97%
3.	Abortion not experienced	211	56.12%	107	72.79%	318	60.80%
4.	Issueless	43	11.43%	21	14.29%	64	12.23%
	Total	376	100%	147	100%	523	100%

Attitude Towards Family Planning

Population explosion has been a baffling problem in India since the time of independence. The problem of rapid population growth is more serious in rural areas and in downtrodden classes, and in slums in urban areas, because of the illiteracy, poverty and ignorance among these classes at one side and the lack of efficiency and commitment of government sources at the other.

In the present study, the awareness and use of family planning devices by the women of rural areas of Uttaranchal Pradesh, the assessment could not be drawn much reliable as the information received through intensive interview by the project director was contradictory to that of through collected data. The data in this regard is shown in tables 6.1, 6.2 and 6.3, reveal that out of 523 married women, 399 (76.29%) have reported that they are aware of the utility of family planning programme, 124 (23.71%) answered in negative. Regarding initiative, only 36 (9.02%) have told that they themselves take initiative in using the devices of family planning 17 (4.26%) have reported that their husbands take initiative in this regard, 346 (86.72%) have reported that both of them use devices of family planning.

TABLE 6.1

Information on use of Family Planning Measure by Respondents

Sl.No.	*Use of Family Planning Measure*	*Garhwal*		*Kumoun*		*Total*	*%*
		f	*%*	*f*	*%*		
1.	Yes	358	95.21%	41	27.89%	399	76.29%
2.	No	18	4.79%	106	72.11%	124	23.71%
	Total	376	100%	147	100%	523	100%

TABLE 6.2

Information on who takes Initiative for Family Planning by Respondents

Sl.No.	*Initiative for Family Planning*	*Garhwal*		*Kumoun*		*Total*	*%*
		f	*%*	*f*	*%*		
1.	Self	6	1.67%	30	73.18%	36	9.02%
2.	Husband	12	3.35%	5	12.19%	17	4.26%
3.	Both	340	94.98%	6	14.63%	346	86.72%
	Total	358	100%	41	100%	399	100%

TABLE 6.3

Information on the Sources of Family Planning Device

Sl.No.	*Sources*	*Garhwal*		*Kumoun*		*Total*	*%*
		f	*%*	*f*	*%*		
1.	Primary Health Centre	74	20.68%	24	58.53%	98	24.56%
2.	Maternity and Child Welfare Centre	86	24.02%	7	17.07%	93	23.31%
3.	Health Visitor (A.N.M.)	90	25.13%	8	19.51%	98	24.56%
4.	Radio, T.V.	92	25.69%	2	4.89%	94	23.56%
5.	N.G.O.	16	4.48%	-		16	4.01%
	Total	358	100%	41	100%	399	100%

But in intensive interviews, several women of Garhwal and Kumoan, both have told that all the husbands are reluctant and neither of them take the risk of minor operation of sterilization (nusbandi) nor they use other devices, for the illusion of weakness and impotency. They force their wives to go through operation or taking pills, which create side effects many times in their whole body system. Only 1.5% educated women told that their husbands co-operated them in this matter.

The sources of information about the utility of family planning in hilly areas are Primary Health Centres, Maternity and Child Welfare Centers, ANM (Anam didi) and NGOs. A few well to do households have radio and T.V. in their houses or in neighbouring houses, so they get information from these sources. The data, in this regard, is shown in table 6.3.

During intensive interviews all the women told that they get contraceptives from Anam Didi and some times from primary health centres. Many times they could not get because of shortage in government's stock. They told that their husbands never purchase 'these things' from the market, although a few educated husbands don't mind and they arrange themselves from Bazaar.

Attitude of women and their family members during pregnancy and after child-birth

Pregnancy period and child-birth is very important and the matter of anxiety for every married couple. For women, the child birth is the matter of life and death, and at the same time the first experience of motherhood is a great pride for every woman. So the pregnancy and child birth is the most crucial issue of woman's reproductive health, so an extra healthcare behaviour and proper medical treatment are needed for this crucial period, But the situation in hilly and tribal areas of Uttaranchal Pradesh is critical for pregnant women, due to some geographical and cultural reasons.

The precautions and medical care during pregnancy in the present study is shown in tables 7.1 to 7.8.

Table 7.1 indicates that 479 (91.59%) women have reported that they take special care during pregnancy and only 44 (8.41%) have told that they do not take special care. Table 7.2 indicates that 112 (21.41%) take nutritious diet such as milk, ghee and fruits etc during pregnancy, 304 (58.13%) have told that if doctor suggests, then they take tonics also besides nutritious diet, 223 (42.64%) have told that they get regular medical checkup during pregnancy and most of the women 405 (77.44%) have told that they avoid heavy work during those months. Table 7.3 shows the place of delivery. 451 (86.23%) have told that the delivery had taken place in home and only 72 (13.77%) have told that they go in the hospital or nearby nursing home for delivery. Table 7.4 indicates that, only 121 (23.14%) women's deliveries are performed by female doctors, 236 (45.12%) by midwives (ANM) and 166 (31.74%) by elderly women of the household or neighbours or relatives. Table 7.5 indicates the precautions taken after the delivery. 237 (45.32%) have told that after child birth, they take milk, ghee, fruits etc and get special care by the family members. 394 (75.33%) have told that if necessary, then, they take tonics and medicines also side by side the nutritious diet. Only 275 (52.59%) women have told that they take care about the cleanliness and hygienic measures during and after the child birth till 40 days. 144 (27.53%) women told that they get normal diet and normal care during and after child birth, they do not get any special diet or medical care except the seclusion and rest of 15 or 20 days which is ritually necessary.

TABLE 7.1

Information on Precautions and Care taken during Pregnancy by Respondents

Sl.No.	*Precaution Taken*	*Garhwal*		*Kumoun*		*Total*	*%*
		f	*%*	*f*	*%*		
1.	Yes	339	90.16%	140	95.23%	479	91.59%
2.	No	37	9.84%	7	4.77%	44	8.41%
	Total	376	100%	147	100%	523	100%

TABLE 7.2

Information on Type of Precautions and Care taken during Pregnancy by Respondents

Sl.No.	*Type of Precaution*	*Garhwal*		*Kumoun*		*Total*	*%*
		f	*%*	*f*	*%*		
1.	Take Nutritious Food	98	26.6%	14	9.52%	112	21.41%
2.	Tonics	188	50%	116	78.91%	304	58.13%
3.	Regular Medical Check up	112	29.78%	111	75.5%	223	42.64%
4.	Avoidance of Heavy Work	532	93.61%	53	36.05%	405	77.44%
	Total						

TABLE 7.3

Information on Place of Delivery

Sl.No.	*Place of Delivery*	*Garhwal*		*Kumoun*		*Total*	*%*
		f	*%*	*f*	*%*		
1.	Home	315	83.78%	136	92.51%	451	86.23%
2.	Hospital	61	16.22%	11	7.49%	72	13.77%
	Total	376	100%	147	100%	523	100%

TABLE 7.4

Information related to who perform Delivery of Respondents

Sl.No.	*Performer of Delivery*	*Garhwal*		*Kumoun*		*Total*	*%*
		f	*%*	*f*	*%*		
1.	Lady Doctor	110	29.26%	11	7.50%	121	23.14%
2.	Midwife	170	45.21%	66	44.89%	236	45.12%
3.	The Elder Ladies	96	25.53%	70	47.61%	166	31.74%
	Total	376	100%	147	100%	523	100%

TABLE 7.5

Information on Precautions taken after Delivery by Respondents

Sl.No.	*Precaution Taken*	*Garhwal*		*Kumoun*		*Total*	*%*
		f	*%*	*f*	*%*		
1.	Use of Fruits, Milk and Ghee etc.	160	42.55%	77	52.38%	237	45.32%
2.	Use of Tonics and Medicine	296	78.72%	98	66.66%	394	75.33%
3.	Special Care about Cleanliness	187	49.73%	88	59.86%	275	52.59%
4.	Nothing Particular	46	12.23%	98	66.66%	144	27.53%
	Total						

TABLE 7.6

Information on Problem related to Child Birth of Respondents

Sl.No.	*Problem Related to Child Birth*	*Garhwal*		*Kumoun*		*Total*	*%*
		f	*%*	*f*	*%*		
1.	Premature Delivery	6	1.59%	2	1.36%	8	1.53%
2.	Excessive Bleeding	15	3.98%	7	4.76%	22	4.21%
3.	Infection (Instrumental)	-	-	-	-	-	-
4.	Infection	-	-	-	-	-	-
5.	Faintness	-	-	-	-	-	-
6.	Weakness	25	6.64%	9	6.12%	34	6.5%
7.	Under Weight Baby	11	2.92%	4	2.72%	15	2.88%
8.	Jaundice, Pneumonia	6	1.59%	2	1.36%	8	1.53%
9.	Early Infant Death	27	7.19%	12	8.17%	39	7.45%
10.	Facing no Major problem only General Weakness	286	76.09%	111	75.5%	397	75.90%
	Total	376	100%	147	100%	523	100%

Table 7.6 indicates the problems related to child birth. Out of 523 married women 8 (1.53%) have experienced the problem of premature delivery, 22 (4.21%) have told that they had to face the problem of excessive bleeding during delivery, 34 (6.5%) had felt too much weakness after child birth, 15 (2.88%) had under-weight babies, 8 (1.53%) told that their new born babies had suffered from jaundice and a few of them pneumonia, and 39 (7.45%) respondents told that they had to suffered the early death of their infants. 397 (75.91%) felt not any major problem but only general weakness.

Table 7.7 indicates the period of rest and resuming the work in the house and outside work after delivery. 281 (53.73%) respondents have reported that they had to do household chores and other work also after the 15 days rest after delivery. 126 (24.09%) have told that they resumed work after one month of delivery, 92 (17.59%) have told that they were fortunate enough and they took rest of 40 days and then they started to work. 24 (4.59%) have told that they had some complications and weakness so they took rest more than 40 days.

TABLE 7.7

Information Related to the Time Taken to Resume work after Delivery of Respondents

Sl.No.	*Time Taken*	*Garhwal*		*Kumoun*		*Total*	*%*
		f	*%*	*f*	*%*		
1.	After 15 Days	134	35.63%	147	100%	281	53.73%
2.	After One Month	126	33.5%	-		126	24.09%
3.	After 40 Days	92	24.48%	-		92	17.59%
4.	More than 40 Days	24	6.39%	-		24	4.59%
	Total	376	100%	147	100%	523	100%

Table 7.8 indicates the pattern of care of new born children during the household chores and out side work. Out of 523 respondents, 61 (11.66%) have told that they themselves

have to manage household work and care of baby side by side and when they had to go outside for the purpose of bringing water or fuel they had to take their babies with them. 413 (78.97%) have reported that their in-laws take care of new born, while they work in or out of house. 49 (9.37%) have told that they belong to nuclear family and their husbands take care of babies while they work.

TABLE 7.8

Information Related Looking After Child during is In and Out of Home Work

Sl.No.	*Who Look after Child*	*Garhwal*		*Kumoun*		*Total*	*%*
		f	*%*	*f*	*%*		
1.	Carry Child with themselves	38	10.10%	23	15.65%	61	11.66%
2.	In-Laws look after baby	298	79.27%	115	78.23%	413	78.97%
3.	Husband take care	40	10.63%	9	6.12%	49	9.37%
	Total	376	100%	147		523	100%

6

Cultural Beliefs and Religious Practices Associated with Health and Diseases

In most of the rural and tribal India, people have some specific convictions and beliefs regarding the role of super-natural powers in day-to-day life of a person, group or community. These are the product of their specific experience in specific situations, which are beyond of control of human beings such as birth, death, illness, disease, famine, flood, whether, good or bad crops and so on. This belief system is internalized in the process of socialization. Kimball Young (1957) has defined a belief system "as a social product which arises out of the matrix of symbolic interaction. The belief refers to a firm conviction or considered opinion or faith in the truth of religious doctrines." Pokrana K. L. (1994), "Belief is an impression about things, whether good or bad, right or wrong and which have a certain impact on the mind". "Most of the beliefs are so deep rooted and traditional that the society does not try to question the validity of the belief." Ramchandran, & Dharam Lingam T., (1983).

There are many beliefs with regard to causation of various prevalent diseases, found not only in rural areas, but also in urban areas, such as the belief that smallpox was due to goddess Shitla's wrath. Such beliefs have led to formation of certain customs and practices among the people, which became means to seek relief from diseases. In an international conference on 'Primary Health Care and Peoples Movement organized by the Co-ordinating Committee for Primary Health Care (Thailand 1986) had stated that, "popular beliefs concerning health and disease, often have a rational basis, if considered in the context of the particular worldview of those who hold it............ Even if germ theory of disease is accepted, still an explanation as to why only some get disease and others do not, is essential. Explanation for them come from belief in witchcraft, evil spirits, evil eyes, anti-social action or a broken taboo."

The beliefs regarding illness, diseases and their treatment go parallel to the modern medical system of treatment almost in all the villages today.

In the same way the religious and ritual beliefs and practices related to pregnancy, child birth and pre and post natal periods, new borns etc. are also prevalent, even in urban societies also. Many studies reveal that certain religious ceremonies in certain months of pregnancy, special care for the protection of fetus and new born with the help of Pooja and Tantra Mantra or Tabeej are common practices in rural and tribal areas particularly.

In the present study of rural and tribal hilly areas of Uttaranchal Pradesh the information collected through intensive interviews and informal discussions with the women by the project director and the data collected by interview schedules, are not similar in regarding the cultural and religious beliefs and practices to treat illness and diseases or during pregnancy or child birth and so on. The data in table 8.1 & 8.2 show that out of 523 respondents 389 (74.37%) have reported that normally they do not believe in such practices but rarely, some times they perform such ritual practices in very complicated cases. Only 134 (25.63%) have accepted the truth that they believe in religious, magical and ritual factors specifically in pregnancy and child birth. They told that they perform special 'Pooja' prescribed by the priest or 'Sayana'. Many times they go to Ojjha for tantra mantra or tabeej or some magical herbs. Table 8.3 indicates the reasons behind these practices. 39 (29.10%) have told that they perform these activities for safe child birth, 10 (7.46%) told to please the gods and ancestors, 14 (10.45%) have told that to avoid the fear of evil spirits, 51 (38.06%) have told that to avoid the fear and harm which their enemies may do them. 20 (14.93%) have told that they perform Pooja or any other device prescribed by the priest or Sayana for the birth of male child.

TABLE 8.1

Information Related on Religious Activities during Pregnancy or Illness

Sl.No.	*Religious Activities*	*Garhwal*		*Kumoun*		*Total*	*%*
		f	*%*	*f*	*%*		
1.	Yes	102	27.12%	32	21.77%	134	25.63%
2.	Some time, but not in regular practice	274	72.88%	115	78.23%	389	74.37%
	Total	376	100%	147	100%	523	100%

TABLE 8.2

Information Related to the Devices of Religious Practice adopted by the Respondents

Sl.No.	*Devices of Religious Practice*	*Garhwal*		*Kumoun*		*Total*	*%*
		f	*%*	*f*	*%*		
1.	Special Pooja of God	102	100%	32	100%	134	100%
2.	Tantra Mantra and Tabeej	-	-	-	-	-	-
3.	Sacred and Magical Herbs	-	-	-	-	-	-
	Total	102	100%	32	100%	134	100%

TABLE 8.3

Information on Reasons behind Religious Practice during Pregnancy and Illness

Sl.No.	Reasons	Garhwal		Kumoun		Total	%
		f	%	f	%		
1.	Safe Child Birth	34	33.33%	5	15.62%	39	29.10%
2.	To Please Ancestors and God	4	3.92%	6	18.75%	10	7.46%
3.	In Fear of Bad Spirits	12	11.78%	2	6.25%	14	10.45%
4.	To Save from Enemies	44	43.13%	7	21.88%	51	38.06%
5.	In Hope of Male Child	8	7.84%	12	37.5%	20	14.93%
	Total	102	100%	32	100%	134	100%

But in informal and friendly discussion with the project director, all the rural women, even some educated intermediate passed women told that they believe in such practices to cure fatal diseases and for safe pregnancy and safe child birth because they repeatedly experienced the 'miracle' of such beliefs and practices so when a specialist of religion or magic prescribes any device, they perform it with full faith and belief and in most of the cases they get the desired results and then these beliefs become more firm and definite.

7

To Identify the Health Care Delivery System and Availability of Medical Facilities

A strong health care delivery system and the proper availability of medical facilities for the masses are the essential parts of the policies of developing nations to secure the target of Health for all as prescribed by the World Health Organization (WHO 1987).

"Health Care indicates not only medical care but also services for promotion of health, prevention of disease, early diagnosis and rehabilitation." (O.P. Sharma, 2000). Medical professionals have a significant role in the way to developing better systems of health care for all with their specialized knowledge, experience and dedication. The number of health care models, preventive and curative, has been developed in every society for the delivery of health care services to the masses. Among these the prevalent models are public (Government) private and voluntary (NGOs).

In the present study, to assess the present health care delivery system in the rural and tribal hilly areas of Uttaranchal Pradesh, the relevant queries have been shown in the tables 9.1 to 9.12.

The table 9.1 indicates that, out of 600 respondents only 353 (58.83%) have told that there are few medical facilities available in their villages or nearby their villages. 247 (41.17%) have answered in negative. Table 9.2 indicates the distance of these facilities from their residence. 289 (81.86%) have told that these are 1 to 3 km. far away from their residence, 26 (7.36%) have told the distance 4 to 6 km and 38 (10.78%) have told that they have to travel more than six km to avail these facilities which is very difficult task.

TABLE 9.1

Information Related to the Availability of Medical Facilities in or nearby Villages of the Respondents

Sl.No.	*Availability of Medical Facilities*	*Garhwal*		*Kumoun*		*Total*	*%*
		f	*%*	*f*	*%*		
1.	Yes	276	69%	77	38.5%	353	58.83%
2.	No	124	31%	123	61.5%	247	41.17%
	Total	400	100%	200	100%	600	100%

TABLE 9.2

Information Related to Distance of Residence from Available Medical Facilities

Sl.No.	*Distance from Residence*	*Garhwal*		*Kumoun*		*Total*	*%*
		f	*%*	*f*	*%*		
1.	1 – 3	212	76.81%	77	100%	289	81.86%
2.	4 – 6	26	9.42%	-		26	7.36%
3.	6- Above	38	13.77%	-		38	10.78%
	Total	276	100%	77	100%	353	100%

Table 9.3 and 9.4 indicates that only 173 (28.83%) have admitted that Primary Health Centers (PHC) and Maternity Health Centers (MHC) are working in their villages and the distance from their residence is 1 to 3 km while 427 (71.17%) have reported that such centres are non-existent in their villages. They have to go to another Village's and Kasbas or Community Health Centres nearby city.

TABLE 9.3

Information related to the Availability of Primary Health Center and Maternity and Child Welfare Center

Sl.No.	*PHC and MHC*	*Garhwal*		*Kumoun*		*Total*	*%*
		f	*%*	*f*	*%*		
1.	Yes	102	25.5%	71	35.5%	173	28.83%
2.	Not in Village but in Kasbas or nearly City	298	74.5%	129	64.5%	427	71.17%
	Total	400	100%	200	100%	600	100%

TABLE 9.4

Information Related to Distance of PHC and MHC from Residence

Sl.No.	*Distance From Residence*	*Garhwal*		*Kumoun*		*Total*	*%*
		f	*%*	*f*	*%*		
1.	0 – 3	102	100%	71	100%	173	100%
2.	4 – 6	-	-	-	-	-	-
3.	6 - More	-	-	-	-	-	-
	Total	102	100%	71	100%	173	100%

Table 9.5 indicates the type of medical institutions in the area. Out of 600 respondents, only 173 (28.84%) have told that PHC and MHC are working in the villages. 86 (14.33%) respondents have reported that there are private doctors and NGO's (Missionary clinics) are working in their villages only 341 (56.83%) have reported that neither government nor private or NGOs are working in their villages.

TABLE 9.5

Information Related to the type of PHC and Other Institutions

Sl.No.	*Type of PHC and Other Institutions*	*Garhwal*		*Kumoun*		*Total*	*%*
		f	*%*	*f*	*%*		
1.	Government	113	28.25%	60	30%	173	28.84%
2.	Non-Government	67	16.75%	19	9.5%	86	14.33%
3.	Neither Government Nor Private or NGOs in the Village	220	55%	121	60.5%	341	56.83%
	Total	400	100%	200	100%	600	100%

TABLE 9.6

Information Related to the visit of Health Personnels ANM etc. in the Villages of Studied Area

Sl.No.	*Visit of Health Personnels*	*Garhwal*		*Kumoun*		*Total*	*%*
		f	*%*	*f*	*%*		
1.	Weekly	100	25%	32	16%	132	22%
2.	Not Weekly But Some Times	31	7.75%	10	5%	41	6.83%
	Total						

Table 9.6 indicates the frequency of the visits of personnels of PHC and MHC, 132 (22%) respondents have told that ANM Deedi and her assistant visit almost once in a week in the village. 41 (6.83%) have reported that ANM Deedi does not live in the village, and she comes from the city, so she mostly stays at the centre and visits many times monthly and some times twice in a month.

Table 9.7 indicates the medical facilities other than PHC or MHC. 196 (32.6%) respondents have told that private doctors are available in their villages or in neighbouring villages. 40 (6.6%) have told that private nursing homes are working in their villages. 50 (8.33%) have told that they go to Hakim ji for the treatment of minor ailments. 22 (3.66%) have told that pathology labs are also available in their villages, only for blood, urine and stool tests side by side general treatment.

TABLE 9.7

Information on Other Resources Except of Government Health Care System

Sl.No.	*Medical Facilities Other than PHC and MHC*	*Garhwal*		*Kumoun*		*Total*	*%*
		f	*%*	*f*	*%*		
1.	Private Doctors	120	30%	76	38%	196	32.6%
2.	Private Nursing Home	30	7.5%	10	5%	40	6.6%
3.	Hakim	40	10%	10	5%	50	8.33%
4.	Homeopathic Doctor	-	-	-	-	-	-
5.	Pathology Lab	15	3.75%	7	3.5%	22	3.66%
	Total						

Table 9.8 indicates the kind of medical facilities available in government dispensaries or PHC etc. Out of 600 respondents 364 (60.66%) have answered that they get only medicines from

government health centres, 306 (51%) have told that they get injections with medicine if needed so, 278 (46.33) have told that tonics such as vitamins and iron tablets are also available in their village PHC. 113 (18.83) have told that in complicated cases the arrangement of blood is also possible. 70 (11.66%) have told that oxygen cylinder may also be arranged in serious cases. Only 2 (0.33%) have told that Ambulance is available in community health centre and not in PHC. The facility of operation (OT) was absolutely absent in the area.

TABLE 9.8

Information Related to Facilities Available in PHC and MHC or Dispensaries

Sl.No.	*Facilities*	*Garhwal*		*Kumoun*		*Total*	*%*
		f	*%*	*f*	*%*		
1.	Medicines	242	60.5%	122	61%	364	60.66%
2.	Injections	204	51%	102	51%	306	51%
3.	Tonics	202	50.5%	76	38%	278	46.33%
4.	Blood	98	24.5%	15	7.5%	113	18.83%
5.	Oxygen Cylinder	70	17.5%	-	-	70	11.66%
6.	Ambulance	2	0.5%	-	-	2	0.33%
7.	Operation	-	-	-	-	-	-
8.	Apparatus of Operation	-	-	-	-	-	-
	Total						

Table 9.9 indicates the frequency of availability of male doctor in PHC or female doctor in PHC or MHC. Out of 600 respondents only 45 (7.5%) have told that the doctor is available twice, morning, evening (ME) in a day, 311 (51.83%) have told that once in a day (M) 102 (17%) have told that doctor is

available only twice in a week; the pharmacist (Chhote Doctor Sahib) takes care of all the patients, every day. 8 (1.33%) told that doctor is available once in a week, the whole sole incharge is pharmacist (Compounder Saheb). 22 (3.67%) have told some times, and 2 (0.33%) have told that doctor saheb is not available any time. Rest of the 110 (18.33%) have not answered properly.

TABLE 9.9

Information Related to Availability of Doctors in Government Hospitals in the Studied Area

Sl. No.	*Availability of Doctor in Government Hospital*	*Garhwal*		*Kumoun*		*Total*	*%*
		f	*%*	*f*	*%*		
1.	Daily two times (Morning-Evening)	30	7.5%	15	7.5%	45	7.5%
2.	Once in a Day (M)	204	51%	107	53.5%	311	51.83%
3.	Twice in a week (M)	86	21.5%	16	8%	102	17%
4.	Once in a week (M)	4	1%	4	2%	8	1.33%
5.	Some Times	16	4%	6	3%	22	3.67%
6.	No	2	0.5%	-	-	2	0.33%
7.	Not Answered	58	14.5%	52	26%	110	18.33%
	Total	400	100%	200	100%	600	100%

Table 9.10 indicates the ratio of utilization of medical facilities available in government health centers (GHC) by the respondents. Out of 600, 391 (65.17%) have told that they used the medical facilities available in their area and 209 (34.83%) have answered in negative and table 9.11 shows the reasons of not availing the facilities of GHC. The reasons of not going are several. 80 (38.28%) have told that due to careless attitude of government doctors they do not go there, 25 (11.98%) have reported the lack of confidence in govt. doctors as the reason of not going there. 10 (4.78%) have complained the rude behaviour of the personnels of government health centres as the major cause of not going there. 12 (5.74%) have told that whenever

they go, the doctor was not available every time, so they do not go now there. 20 (9.6%) have told that most of the time there is shortage of medicines in the stock of GHC, so there is no use of going there. 62 (29.66%) have told that the distance of GHC is too much long so it is not possible for them to go for the treatment there.

TABLE 9.10

Information Related to the Utilization of Available Health Facilities by the Respondents

Sl.No.	*Utilization of Available Health Facilities*	*Garhwal*		*Kumoun*		*Total*	*%*
		f	*%*	*f*	*%*		
1.	Yes	235	58.75%	156	78%	391	65.17%
2.	No	165	41.25%	44	22%	209	34.83%
	Total	400	100%	200	100%	600	100%

TABLE 9.11

Information Related to the Reasons behind not using Health Facilities by Respondents

Sl.No.	*Reasons behind not using Health Facilities*	*Garhwal*		*Kumoun*		*Total*	*%*
		f	*%*	*f*	*%*		
1.	Carelessness of Government Doctors	65	39.40%	15	34.09%	80	38.28%
2.	Lack of Confidence	18	10.90%	7	15.90%	25	11.98%
3.	Rude Behaviour of Doctors	2	1.2%	8	18.19%	10	4.78%
4.	Absence of Doctors	10	6.06%	2	4.55%	12	5.74%
5.	Absence of Medicines and Facilities	10	6.06%	10	22.72%	20	9.56%
6.	Too Much distance from Home	60	36.38%	2	4.55%	62	29.66%
	Total	165	100%	44	100%	209	100%

Table 9.12 is about the options taken by the respondents in the cases of absence of medical facilities in Govt. PHC or MHC, or government dispensaries, 156 (26%) respondents have told that they go to the private doctor of the village for the treatment, 168 (28%) have told that they go to district hospitals, 97 (16.17%) have told that they go to low-cost small nursing homes, 121 (20.17%) have told that they prefer to go to specialists in the city, if needed. 58 (9.66%) have told that they can afford even costly treatment and they do not like to take risk in the state of illness or diseases, so they go to costly nursing homes, where every modern medical facility is available for emergency.

TABLE 9.12

Information Related to the Options used by the Respondents in place of Government Health Facilities in Studied Area

Sl.No.	*Option used in place of Government Health Facilities*	*Garhwal*		*Kumoun*		*Total*	*%*
		f	*%*	*f*	*%*		
1.	Private Doctor of Village	110	27.5%	46	23%	156	26%
2.	District Hospitals	102	25.5%	66	33%	168	28%
3.	Nursing Home	65	16.25%	32	16%	97	16.17%
4.	Specialist of Cities	80	20%	41	20.5%	121	20.17%
5.	Costly Nursing Home of Cities	43	10.75%	15	7.5%	58	9.66%
	Total	400	100%	200	100%	600	100%

8

To Identify the Pattern of Social Relationships and Social Support System

Man is a social animal. The personality of every individual is the outcome of the process of interaction and socialization which occurs in a definite set of socio-cultural system. The patterns of social relationships with family members, Kith and Kin, neighbours, friends and other primary and secondary groups are the important factors in determining the mental and physical health of persons. David, Brunner and Wilkinson (1996) have opined that "each population of people is immersed in a social milieu. The social milieu has dozen of features that are important to health." The latest approach to the health problem of communities and societies which has commanded growing recognition among the modern experts of medical profession is the socio ecological approach which assumes that the health of the people is predominantly the net result of the interaction of people with their social milieu. "In this context many sociological work has explored the relationship between peoples health and their interactive social network." Steve Taylor and David Field (2003).

This approach is the reaction to the ultra modern industrial mass society's way of living which is named by the social scientists as the "world of tenuous and loosely knitted social relationships." 'Stress and strains' have been described as the epidemic of such modern societies. A number of studies have shown that "stressful life-style can make people more vulnerable to disease and even premature death." Taylor & Field (2003). The medical experts of today, have realized the fatal consequences of constantly decreasing intensity and warmth of human ties and weakening relationships among family and kinship members which are responsible for creating new complicated mental health problems in the masses. More than a century ago, Durkheim (1952) in his theory of suicide has established that the more people are integrated into the social groups around them, the less vulnerable they are to suicide. A study by Berkman and Syme (1979) revealed that, "the persons who were married, had regular contact with friends and relatives, had church membership and membership of voluntary organizations, among them the percentage of morbidity and mortality was three times lesser than among those who were poorly integrated and isolated." The researchers opined that "social support provided by integration, is beneficial in promoting health and its major benefit is as a buffer in helping people cope with stressful life experiences." Taylor & Field (2003).

Nyamathi (et al 2000) has found in a study of homeless women that among drug addicted patients, those were more likely to be receptive to drug treatment programme, who had social support than those who had no support. Taylor & Field (2003) have observed that, "Social Support operates at different levels–'Emotional Support', which can reassure the patients that they are still cared, 'Instrumental Support', such as physical care, financial help, help in child care or shopping etc. 'Informational Support', such as information about good doctor, proper diet, or about other precautions." Modern medical professionals have treated the 'Social Support System', as a significant instrument in recovery from illness, even in fatal diseases such as depression, heart disease and cancers etc.

It is obvious from the above discussion that social support system has a tremendous role in healing the illness and re-establish the sense of self-esteem and recovery from depression in the patients. It is a fascinating paradox of modern times, that rapid growth of economic prosperity and industrialization, the urban societies are loosing the social support system due to constant weakening of bondage of primary social relationships, while the rural communities, despite their poverty and deprivation from modern facilities of life, they belong to a strong social support system due to integrated interrelationship and emotional ties and 'we' feeling among the members within the communities.

In the present study the picture of social support system is very bright and the situation is encouraging and optimistic as the data shown in the tables 10.1 to 10.4, collected from the respondents of rural and hilly areas of Uttaranchal Pradesh.

TABLE 10.1

Information on Type of Relationships with Relatives of the Respondents

Sl.No.	*Type of Relations with Relatives*	*Garhwal*		*Kumoun*		*Total*	*%*
		f	*%*	*f*	*%*		
1.	Good	390	97.5%	187	93.5%	577	96.17%
2.	Neutral	9	2.25%	13	6.5%	22	3.67%
3.	Bad	1	0.25%	-	-	1	0.16%
	Total	400	100%	200	100%	600	100%

TABLE 10.2

Information on Which Kind of Help in Crisis Respondents Get

Sl.No.	*Kind of Help in Crisis*	*Garhwal*		*Kumoun*		*Total*	*%*
		f	*%*	*f*	*%*		
1.	Money	275	68.75%	174	87%	449	74.83%
2.	By taking Doctors	252	63%	147	73.5%	399	66.5%
3.	In Nursing of Patient	267	66.75%	182	91%	449	74.83%
4.	Help in Household	284	71%	134	67%	418	69.66%
5.	Looking after of children in case of Illness or any other calamity	223	55.75%	117	58.5%	340	56.66%
	Total						

Table 10.1 indicates the pattern of relationships of respondents with their relatives and table 10.2 indicates the kind of help, which they get from their kiths and kins at the time of crisis, specifically at the time of illness, child birth or any other calamity. Out of 600 respondents, 577 (96.17%) have informed that they have very good relations with their relatives, only 22 (3.67%) have reported that neither good, nor bad but neutral relations they have with their relatives and only 1 (0.16%) has reported that her family has not good relations with relatives due to an old enemity. Table 10.2 indicates that a high degree of cooperation is found among the rural and tribal community's inhabitants at the time of crisis. The table shows that out of 600 respondents 449 (74.83%) have informed that their relatives render every kind of help including financial help at the time of illness or any other emergency. 399 (66.5%) have reported that their relatives help them in taking medical help such as calling for doctor, bringing medicines from market or taking to hospital etc. 449 (74.83%) have told that at the time of illness or delivery in the house, their relatives help them

in nursing the patients including other kinds of help. 418 (69.66%) have told that their relatives help them in household work side by side with other kinds of help. 340 (56.66%) have told that their relatives co-operate them in looking after of children at the time of illness or child birth.

TABLE 10.3

Information Related to the type of Relations with Neighbours of the Respondents

Sl.No.	*Kind of Relations with Neighbors*	*Garhwal*		*Kumoun*		*Total*	*%*
		f	*%*	*f*	*%*		
1.	Good	362	90.5%	182	91%	544	90.67%
2.	Neutral	26	6.5%	18	9%	44	7.33%
3.	Not Good	12	3%	-		12	2%
	Total	400	100%	200	100%	600	100%

TABLE 10.4

Information on which Kind of Help, Respondents Get from the Neighbour in Crisis

Sl. No.	*Kind of Help in Crisis*	*Garhwal*		*Kumoun*		*Total*	*%*
		f	*%*	*f*	*%*		
1.	Help in going to Doctor	223	55.75%	119	59.5%	342	57%
2.	Help in Nursing at Home	198	49.5%	146	73%	344	57.33%
3.	Financial Help	258	64.5%	159	79.5%	417	69.5%
4.	Limited to Formal Inquiries about Illness or any other calamity	24	6%	34	17%	58	9.66%
	Total						

The tables 10.3 and 10.4 show the pattern of relations with the neighbours in the hilly rural and tribal areas of

Uttaranchal Pradesh. Out of 600 respondents, 544 (90.66%) have told that they have very good relations with their neighbours and they are always co-operative in day to day matters and at the time of crises or illness, they render every kind of help, if they can afford, such as carrying to the doctor for treatment, nursing at home, help with money and material and looking after the children if needed so. Only 44 (7.33%) respondents told that they have formal relations with their neighbours only limited to formal inquiries about health or any other calamity. 12 (2%) have reported that their relations with neighbours are not good.

9

Analysis and Conclusion

Part – I

Introduction

This research project presents a sociological analysis of one of the myriad burning issues related to womankind which is not important for the life and existence of woman herself only, but essentially, related to the existence of whole humanity, society and nation's life, and the issue is – 'The Medical and Health Care of Women' with special reference to their 'Reproductive Health'. For convenience, the present study can be summarized as follows.

The first part of chapter-I, introduces the subject matter, statement of problem, significance and relevance of the study. In the Second part of chapter-I, a systematic review of related studies has been discussed in order to get an overview of the present status of knowledge related to the subject of research, so that the objectives and universe of the study may help to cover the areas of research and knowledge, which are untouched and unexplored yet. At the same time for the guidance of research work, a few hypotheses were formulated.

In the last part of this chapter, the concepts, which were used in the study, have been explained to make for better understanding.

Problem and Perspective

The health issue of womenfolk, during last some decades, is gaining more and more concern with the scholars of various disciplines. An issue, which has so many significant implications on the national and social life of the masses, such as continuous decreasing proportion of women in India's population since 1901 census, high female infant mortality rate, increasing trend of female foeticide, week physique and low efficiency level of new generations etc. It is but natural for a student of sociology to go deep into the subject and to enquire the ground reality beneath the layers. Thus the researcher has made an humble attempt to study the problem of medical and health care of women with the help of a micro-field-study of some of the hilly and tribal areas of Uttaranchal Pradesh.

Although, health is generally considered a bio-medical phenomenon, and illness and diseases are treated with bio-medical approach. But with the emergence of medical sociology and the modern humane approach to the health problems, it is vastly admitted and accepted that health of an individual or community is a complex phenomenon, which is largely influenced by social and cultural factors.

The interrelationship between illness and health and a given social situation is not entirely new to the field of sociology. Right from the pioneer social thinkers like Hippocrate, Durkheim, Ogburn, Spencer to modern social thinkers like Parsons, Wilson, Hawkins and others directly or indirectly stated illness and disease as a social phenomenon and suggested the social environment as an etiological factor in disease and illness and emphasized doctor-patient relationship as a therapeutic tool.

In the light of above discussion, it may fairly become justified that there is vast scope for the student of sociology to study the health problem of any social group, segment or community at large. Present endeavour, in the form of research Project, took the courage to understand this complex social problem of women-folk.

Now the question arises that what is the importance of health for a person ! The answer to this question could not be understood better than through that mythological episode described in the great epic 'Mahabharata', in which Yaksha asked the eldest Pandava brother Yudhishthira "लाभानामुत्तमं किं स्यात्" ? (What is the most precious thing in the world for human happiness ?) The wise Dharmraj Yudhishthira answered "लाभानाम् श्रेयः आरोग्यम्". (The most precious thing in the world for human happiness is a disease free healthy body with health mind.) Singhi and Pokrana (1994) also stated that "in ancient Greece as well as in India, health was conceived man's precious possession and was treated as a cherished goal of life."

If health was realized the most precious treasure of life in ancient age, it is as much precious in modern, scientific age as well. Eminent economist Whipple observed that "A nation's true wealth is not in its land and waters, not in its flocks and herds, not in its treasure of dollars, but in its healthy and happy men, women and children." (Whipple, 2001)

Here, it should be mentioned that although the specific purpose of this study is 'The Medical and Health Care of Women', but for the student of sociology it is impossible to alienate any human problem from its socio-cultural context and to study it in an absolute manner, specially of women's health which is totally the outcome of socio-cultural setup of any society, modern or traditional. So an humble attempt has been made for better understanding to analyze the health problem of women relative to the status and role of woman in family and society at large.

Women and Society

Although, demographically women constitute half of the humanity, but in the real sense, she is the creator of whole of the humanity. Due to her anatomy and distinctive feminine qualities, nature has imposed on her the burden of gestation, parturition and lactation of the child, who is the source of evolution of human race. The bearing and rearing of the child is the wholesole responsibility of the mother. She is the main agency of socialization of new generations in the family or the household.

Besides these indispensable duties, women of today from educated middle and upper-middle strata of society, are making appreciable contribution in many intellectual, technical and professional fields of 'Nation Building'.

It is really unfortunate for the nation and society, that women resource, which constitute nearly 50 percent of the total Human Resource, has been deprived of its self respect, education, adequate medical care, health, food and nutrition, economic and political participation after 58 years of independence of the nation. She is denied even the right to birth and life till recently.

Health and Women

In women's case the health issue is not merely a medical or physical phenomenon, but it is a complex social phenomenon. It is emphatically stated in the C.S.W.I. report (1974) that, "for women, health is both an important factor in the achievement of status as well as the indicator of social status, because it is conditioned to a great extent by social attitudes of society."

After the survey of long three years period, 'The Commission on the Status of Women' reported that, "All the available evidence leads us to conclude that high female mortality rate and decreasing female ratio after every census is due to the consistent neglect of Female Health." (C.S.W) (1974, p. 312).

After independence, although the Government of India has made considerable efforts to initiate and implement the health policies for women and children, such as to formulate 'separate division' in planning commission for women and children, in 1978, "Health for All by 2000 AD", in 1983, to enact comprehensive health policy which has enunciated the long term demographic goals and other selected time bound programmes to elevate the health status of masses.

But if we compare the progress of health policies, programmes and their implementation in terms of the people's needs, the overall picture of rural areas, tribal areas and slums in the urban areas, remain dismal in the country.

So there seems to be a vicious-circle of poverty and Health problem in the backward, down trodden and weaker sections of society vis a vis to national scenario. This complicated national problem needs to be tackled seriously.

As a remedial effort, to lessen this major problem of the country, a committed class of Social Scientists, Anthropologists and Research Oriented Personnels, can contribute a lot in generating relevant information of various micro-groups and communities or societies by scientific investigation. They may prepare data profile, may analyze reports and they may render valuable suggestions based on the felt needs of the people, which may be very much useful for policy makers, National Planners and other relevant agencies, established by the Government for the task.

It is hoped that the analysis and the findings of the present study "The Medical and Health Care of Women" Living in 'Rural and Tribal Hilly Regions of Uttranchal Pradesh', will make contribution in the realm of research and knowledge and also may be used for making proper policies and programmes to elevate the health status of the vulnerable sections of society.

Review of Literature

The pioneering and independent studies on various aspects and problems of women's lives received vast importance in post independence era in India and after the World War II in countries abroad. Some studies concentrated on such aspects of women's lives as marriage and family, education, exploitation of women, politics and religion etc. Some of them are on the issues like women's participation in the unskilled; skilled and professional jobs and their problems of role conflict.

A class of Sociologists, Educationists, Anthropologists and the Scholars of Medical Science had written a lot in the field of medical and health in India and abroad.

A brief discussion and main findings of those researches, books and reports is presented, which have been directly or indirectly found useful in the formulation of the hypotheses and in selecting the problem and area of the present study.

After the Critical evaluation of existing literature in the field of medical and health sociology in India, specially regarding women's health, attempts made so far suffer from the many significant limitations.

Apart from many other limitations, the fact remains that none of these studies has taken interest in researching women's health problems in the Rural and Tribal Hilly Areas of Uttaranchal Pradesh. The reason may be, that it is a newborn state, which came into existence only in November (2000). Previously it was a part of a huge state- Uttar Pradesh and was neglected because of its Hilly and complicated Geographical conditions. So it had fairly hypothesized that this area of study is unexplored, untraversed and uninvestigated; so the present endeavour made an humble effort to go deep into the ground reality regarding medical and health care of women living in Hilly Areas of Uttaranchal Pradesh.

The Present Study

The problem under taken in this project is to study the status and condition of tribal and rural women of hilly areas of Uttaranchal Pradesh, who are the deprived classes of the society. The project is concentrated mainly on the socio-economic profile of the women, their social status and role in the family, their health condition, the attitude of women towards their own health care, specifically towards their reproductive health. At the same time it has thrust upon the study of public health care system, health facilities available in the area, the attitude of women to take benefit of health facilities available in the area, the attitude of male and female members of the family towards the health care of women in the household. The role of NGO's, if any, in generating health consciousness among women and efforts made by these NGOs regarding health measures in this region, have been also taken in the study. And finally, the pattern of social relationships with the relatives and neighbours has been inquired.

The Relevance of the Study

The present study is targeted to health problem of rural and tribal women living in hilly areas of Uttaranchal Pradesh for the following reasons:-

First - Many rural and tribal communities are living in isolated or semi-isolated areas of hills and forests where modern facilities of medical and health care are not available or partially available. So it is the matter of concern to know how they face the situation at the time of health crises.

Second - The health matter, in remote hilly areas of rural and particularly in tribal groups, is, as such a function of the interaction between socio-cultural and socio-biological practices, food habits and nutritional status, the genetic attributes and the environmental conditions, use of herbal drugs, taboos and superstitions which make the health system very much complicated in that areas, which should be studied from socio-analytical point of view.

Third - The hilly region of Garhwal is inhibited by a tribe (Khasa) of Jaunsar Bawar Region, known for its typical family and marriage custom 'polyandry' which has direct and indirect effects on women's health and demographic balance.

Fourth - Women are the backbone of domestic life, main agency of socialization of new generations. At the same time, women are major part of labour force in the rural and tribal areas of Uttaranchal Pradesh. So their health status must be evaluated.

Fifth - And finally at the last but not the least the health issue of women has multifarious repercussions on the personality and status of women and also on the various aspects of nation's life.

Keeping all the above facts in view, the researcher has decided to investigate the phenomenon of 'women's health status' in hilly areas of Uttaranchal Pradesh.

The Objectives and the hypotheses of the study have been discussed in Chapter-I (see page 45-46)

Conceptual Framework

Various concepts are used in this study. These have been briefly explained in the following paragraphs.

Medical Care

The term medical care denotes the "Science or practice of the diagnosis, treatment and prevention of disease." (Oxford Dictionary). As a profession, medical care means the service rendered by a doctor or physician to develop better system of healthcare for the people in society.

Traditionally, it was considered as a noble profession. A 'Doctor' or a 'Vaidya' was treated as 'Dhanvantri' (The life giver) and was revered next to God by the patients and their relatives. The spirit of service and altruism were prominent than the value of money or wealth. But now it has become a commercial industry with high profit motive.

Health

Generally, health implies a state of sound and fit body with sound mind, which is able to adapt with the physical environment. But from sociological point of view, health does not mean simply a disease free state of the body, but it is a social phenomenon. As stated by World Health Organization (WHO) "Health is a state of complete physical, mental and social well being and not merely the absence of disease and infirmity." (Preamble to constitution of WHO, 1948).

Health Care includes not only medical care, but also services for promotion of health, prevention of disease, early diagnosis and rehabilitation.

Woman

"The female sex in the species of human race" (Oxford Dictionary). Woman is generally known to be contextually identified in India as being a daughter, wife and mother. Encyclopaedia Britanica put the concept in this manner "The very word woman sums up a long history of dependence and subordination." The great historian Gibbon stated that according to ancient law, the woman - a sex created to please and to obey was never supposed to have attained the age of reason. (Kidwai 1978)

According to the constitution of India "women - a weaker section of society - deserving special protection, care and welfare."

Now, after the declaration of Women's Development Decade by the U.N.O, by and large, women are theoretically called as the co-partners in the development process of every country.

Status and Role

Every society is a network of statuses and respective roles. Sociologists and Anthropologists defined 'status' "The place in a particular system, which a certain individual occupies at a particular time, will be referred to as his status with respect to that system." (Linton)

Elliott and Merrill stated that, "Status is the position which an individual occupies in the group by virtue of his sex, age, family, occupation, marriage and achievement."

In sociological literature woman's status is often used as a synonym for 'role'. According to Majumdar and Madan " actual treatment, legal status, opportunity for social participation and the character and extent of work, all determine each as a specific sense and manner, the status of women in a society."

In woman's case her status and role in society is determined by social and conventional expectations than her role in economic participation.

Public Health care Delivery System

Health Care Delivery System denotes the health care services provided by the government agencies free of cost. It includes not only medical curative measures but also services for promotion of health, prevention of diseases and epidemics and other measures taken in the sphere of hygiene , sanitation and to reduce pollution and other ecological problems.

N.G.O.s

By its original meaning, "A voluntary organization was a grouping of volunteers joined together with shared value of concerned for a specific goal. The main purpose was to render welfare service to the needy and depressed people." This has been selfless and unpaid service to humanity. But this type of welfare activities is now a gone history.

Today, N.G.O. (Non Governmental organizations) consist of full-time paid trained staff of social workers, as well as committed professionals from many fields, who believe in the specific 'cause' to which they devote their time as a full time activity. (Desai A.S. 1998)

Research Design

Chapter II presents research design keeping in view the problem, perspective and objectives of the present study (See Chapter I).

The quest for novelty is eternal in man. The mysteries of cosmic phenomena have been the fascinating matter of man's curiosity from time immemorial. In the process of exploring and understanding, he has tried to know the causal-relations among the various events-natural or human, and draw the conclusions to reach the realm of truth and reality. The scholars of natural and social-sciences called this process of learning, exploring and understanding the truth and reality–'The Scientific Method'. Present study 'The Medical and Health-Care of Women in the Hilly and Tribal Regions of Uttaranchal Pradesh' in the form of major project research work has also tried to follow the scientific method, tools and techniques and tried to its best tó maintain the objectivity in the whole process in order to find out the truth and reality.

The purpose of the present study is to explore and evaluate the health status of rural and tribal women of Uttaranchal Pradesh, so, some relevant objectives and a few hypothesis were set properly. (See Chapter I).

Area of the Study

The researcher has taken the two districts, Dehradun & Almora of Uttaranchal State as the Universe of The Study, because after reviewing the literature, it came to be notice that none of these studies had taken interest in finding out women's health problems in Hilly areas of Uttaranchal Pradesh.

The selection of Dehradun Distt. (Jaunsar Bawar Area) and Almora (Kumoun Region) was purposive. The study of Jaunsar Bawar is of special interest to the sociologists, because it is inhabited by the 'Khasa Tribe', who has followed different religio-social system and the custom of polyandry. The research hypothesised that this custom might have influenced the health and fertility of the women in this area. Researcher has selected Almora district because of its remoteness, poverty, backwardness and lack of modern facilities.

Sampling Frame

The whole process of sampling, which is adopted for the present study is Purposive, Stratified and Random depending upon the nature and objectives of the study.

Techniques of Data Collection

In this study the following techniques were adopted for data collection –

(i) Interview Schedule

An interview schedule, based on the main objectives of the study was formulated.

(ii) Intensive Interview and Observation

To verify the facts and cross check the information supplied by the investigators through interview schedules, and moreover to make the study and research work more reliable, the project director carried out intensive field survey of the area with the help of Surpanch, Panchayat members and social workers of the regions under study.

(iii) Collective Interview and Focus Interview

With the help of women panchayat members and social workers, the group interview were also organized in the local temple campus and at the residence of sarpanch also.

(iv) Case Studies

On the basis of individual intensive interviews with some respondents, doctors, ANMs and NGOs, a few case studies have been prepared, which are mentioned in appendix 1 in the report.

(v) Additional Aids to Data Collection

To make the study more objective and realistic, the researcher has used camera and tape-recorder.

(vi) Secondary Sources of Data Collection

Census Reports, Maps, Journals and Relevant Books from various libraries were also used to make the study more informative.

Processing of Data

After the collecting all 600 interview schedules and completing the intensive field survey, the informations were tabulated mechanically to find out the results.

Interpretation and Analysis

On the basis of data, several tables were designed to find out the information and conclusions. The results were compared across the hypotheses of the study.

Findings and Suggestions

A summary of the whole report and findings were presented. Some suggestions were given which might be used to lessen the health hazards of women living in remote hilly areas.

Limitations of the Study

The study had been concerned with the health problems of women living in remote hilly and tribal villages of Dehradun and Almora districts, specifically from poor and downtrodden classes. Thus the conclusions drawn from this study may not be applicable to the women from economically well to do households and women, living in Urban Areas of Uttaranchal Pradesh.

It is an academic venture and purely empirical and exploratory sociological analysis, based on the facts obtained through schedules, observations and intensive interviews. The interpretation of facts and data had been done as far as possible objectively, subject to the constraints of human error.

However, an humble effort had been made to present the true picture of women's health hazards in remote hilly and tribal areas with the hope that the analysis and findings may be used for making proper health policies and programmes to elevate the Health Status of women.

Socio-economic Profile of the Respondents

In the Chapter III, Socio-economic profile had been discussed. It provides the base for any enquiry of groups, classes or communities. The identity of a person is recognized through his or her status and role in the system of social structure.

For the present study, to assess the health behaviour of rural and tribal women of Uttaranchal Pradesh, such components of socio-economic status as age, marital status, caste, religion, family pattern, educational level, occupational background, sources of income etc. have been realized relevant for enquiry. (See Chapter III)

After processing and analyzing the whole data, the researcher found that majority of the respondents belonged to the **age** in between 18 to 45, which is most fertile and most crucial as regards the health and child bearing period. Women in hills, generally get married before the age of 18 and then they bear the responsibility of the whole household side by side child bearing and rearing even till the age of 55.

Regarding health, it came to notice during collective interviews, that most of the women of this age group had the problems like backache, anemia and irregular periods. Some of them were lactating mothers, their faces were pale and they seemed tired, still they don't take extra nutrition and never said that they were sick. They do their routine work (in and out of home). These problems are part and parcel of day to day life for these young daughters in-law. The most privileged classes are boys, husbands and mothers in-law in the matter of health-care.

Regarding **religion** there seems no disparity as all respondents followed Hinduism according to collected data. But during intensive field survey by the project director, an educated Christian family came into contact.

Regarding the **relationship between religion and health**, religion plays an important role in the treatment of diseases in rural and tribal societies.

During intensive interview, even those women, who were educated upto intermediate classes, have expressed the faith on healers who use rituals, religion and magic for healing of such type of patients, which were not cured by the doctors or the patients of some unknown diseases.

Caste is still a dominant factor in the disparities about the Health and Cleanliness standard of the women folk. Majority of women of the sample belonged to the general categories of the so-called high castes but a good percentage belonged to the scheduled caste also. The Scheduled Tribes were mainly confined to the area of Chakarata in Dehradun. During intensive interview, it was observed by the project director that high caste women were more health conscious than low caste's women. But Tribal (Jaunsari) women were also health conscious because of their better economic conditions and high caste status.

The level of education is not depressing, as 60% women were educated upto primary and high school and they were mostly above 30. The highly educated number of women was very tiny. But the new generation was coming forward in this field and it was found that nearly all the daughters of the family were being sent to school. Regarding health matters, education does not play a significant role as the study reveals that even less or uneducated women were also health conscious if they were of high caste or from the better economic class.

Marriage is still an important institution in the remote hilly region and is considered the only goal of woman's life. Early marriage before the age of 18 was found to be common. In the sample selected, most of the women interviewed were married (80%), those unmarried were young girls, there was hardly a case of divorce or remarriage. A divorce single woman is rare in the hills but unofficially deserted women are quite common in these regions. Among the respondents, there were a few cases of widows who never remarried, but ever they stayed with their sons or nephew's families and performed all the household duties. In Kumaon region, inter caste marriages are still unknown, but marriage itself is not such a serious problem in these areas and daughters are not supposed to be a burden. The problem of dowry is non existent as the researcher tried to find through personal interviews. But the impact of urban culture is slowly entering these regions. The rural urban continuam is negatively affecting this institution and the so called educated families are demanding dowry and the torture of daughters in-law has started showing its impact.

The structure of family, in most of the Hindu villages, is still joint, although joint family means three or more generations living together. Most of the families of Kumaon and Garhwal are still bound with their lands – which is the most important binding force. They have their own houses, whether Kachas or Puccas, and being emotionally attached to their land of ancestors, they do not want to move out of their villages. This might be the reason for the prevalence of joint families in these regions. But even the percentage of Nuclear families is no less (41.3%). The concept of single mothers is non existent single father & children is also a rare phenomenon.

As far as the **occupational status and the earning capacity** is concerned, it is strange that women share the double responsibility of looking after the house and children in the morning and then moving out of house to go into the fields (to cut the grass or to look after the crop). Even caring of the cattle is also their duty. This of course tells upon their health. The main source of income of these families is from agriculture. Some families also get income from the cattle breeding; some of them were laborers, maids or vendors also. In short, these hilly communities are still dependent on the flora and fauna of the hills for their survival.

The only security that these people have, is of the **residence**. Nearly all of them have their own houses-whether kuccha or pucca. As far as the **location of houses** is concerned, it is really very sad that there are still no proper means of transport and people have to walk mile after mile on the hilly tracks. This present a great obstacle- for example – the health centers and doctor's clinics are located at distances of many kilometers and patients have to be carried on foot. In case of emergencies the patient is carried on either shoulders, Cot or Doli. These are some serious practical difficulties in the remote hilly areas. Due to natural surroundings in these hilly regions, ventilation is no problem in these houses – they have plenty of sun and air.

In short, it can be fairly estimated from the available data that half of the households are living in below the poverty line, and another one third also live in poverty and hard economic conditions. They have land, but very small (uneconomic holdings). So both men and women, specially women have to do hard work to pull on the family's expenses, because men of hills (both in Kumoun and Garhwal) are mostly habitual of drinking cheap wines and other alcoholic drugs and side by side, they kill their whole day in playing cards. The total burden of the household, whether domestic chores or to earn money, is on the shoulders of the women. Despite of hard labour, researcher was informed (during intensive interview) by women, that wife battering by drunkard husbands is the fate of 80 to 90% women, of these hilly regions.

Health Indicators of Respondents

In Chapter IV, some important aspects of behavior related to health, such as personal hygiene, food habits, general condition of physical health, capacity and duration of working hours, attitude and awareness towards their health-care, attitude towards cleanliness during monthly periods are discussed in detail. (see chapter IV)

But all of these indicators are related to the socio cultural and environmental factors. For example the availability of water determines whether the women take bath, wash clothes, wash their hair daily or once a weak. Among the respondents, it was found that daily bath is not common (only 32%) and mostly women bathe twice a week. Washing of hair daily is not possible. However, the women are well aware of the cleanliness of teeth, nails.

Maintenance of cleanliness during the periods, is a part of religious beliefs. Some taboos are still observed and if a woman breaks the rule, the gods will be displeased and the whole community will suffer for it – in the form of any natural or social calamity – disease, death, or even children going astray. The age old practice of washing the cloth and using it again and again is still prevalent. Only a few young girls belonging to a comparatively higher economic status, made use of sanitary Napkins. The acute shortage of water, heavy snowfall in winter and poverty might be responsible in the lack of hygienic measures.

Inspite of knowing the importance of proper, balanced food, the women of this region seem to be very casual about their food. Some cook just once in a day, while twice a day is the common practice. Most commonly grown cereal in this region is the Macca and Rice and people use it in abundance. Breakfast is not common. The morning meals by 10 a.m. and the evening meals at night and in between, these women work in the fields. Distinction between the vegetarian and non-vegetarian food is not much marked and most of the families are vegetarian. The intake of tea is quite common, while the use of wine by the males is the serious socio-economic and ethical issue for the women. Fruits and vegetables are luxury because even if they grow themselves, they sell in the market to get some extra income.

So, it was found, after personal observation, that the women were undernourished. Some of the young women, who were feeding their babies, had pale yellow cheeks, with no special nourishment during pregnancy or lactation.

Strangely enough, it was found that few or none of the women complained much about their general physical condition i.e. pain in the legs, backache, tiredness and breathlessness were supposed to be a part of normal health system and unless a woman is bed ridden, she is not supposed to be sick. She goes to work in the field just after a week or two weeks of delivery. They must go to fetch water from anywhere for cooking and other domestic purposes despite of their illness, because no male of the house would ever do that – and they must not complain. Similarly, they must give a lion's share of the food to their husbands and eat the left over, otherwise they are not good wives and are criticized. Some foods are prohibited for the feeding mother like bananas, ghee or rich food etc. due to some prevailing superstitions. All these facts came into light only during focus interview with the project director.

With the exception of girl child and very old women, the women of these regions work for more than four to eight hours in the fields – not to mention the household work they finish before going out. The day begins early in the morning, with hardly any rest and ends at night. The elderly women look after the infants and children.

In the matter of care and precaution during illness, it was noticed during survey that in initial stage of sickness, most of the women seemed reluctant to go to the doctor and prefer to take home made herbal medicines like Tulsi, Haldi, Oil massage etc. In case of serious medical problems, these women go to the cities to private doctors as most of the women gave a very negative picture of the government doctors or PHCs. The medicines prescribed are not available and they have to purchase from the market. This fact was also verified by the personal interviews. The doctors also informed that important medicines were not available in the dispensary. Only Iron Tablets & Vitamins are supplied. It has been generally observed that the women folk are not satisfied with the behaviour of the staff and facilities provided by the government.

To Identify the Reproductive Behaviour of Women

In chapter V, to assess the reproductive behaviour of women, a comprehensive range of factors such as attitude towards marriage, number of children, attitude towards family planning measures, precautions taken during pregnancy, attitude towards abortion, medical care during pre and post natal periods, source and place of child birth, period of rest and care after child birth, care of infant and so on were inquired through interview schedules and personal interviews by the project director also.

A safe motherhood, and a healthy normal child is one of the fundamental rights of a woman. In the traditional societies, pregnancy, child birth are supposed to be part of natural phenomenon and therefore, for years, women treat child birth as a natural process. Most of the respondents got married by the age of 18 years. A few of them were married even between 20 – 25. To remain single or unmarried is not common. There are no particular criteria for marriage –only woman as a wife, is required to look after the household and also work in fields or jungles for fuel. So it was felt that there is no emotional or moral basis of marriage. Sex-education is not given formally to the girls before marriage but they seem to get to know about it from their surroundings. The researcher had a deep interview with girl students of class IX on the subject. They all were against of early marriage. Generally, there is no bias on the gender basis in the family and the girls are given equal status but as a daughter-in-law, she is totally under sub-ordination of her mother-in-law and husband. About the number of children, the decision is taken, either by the in-laws or by the husbands. Most of the families had on average 3 to 4 children. On asking whether the desire for a male child had affected the number of children, the response was not very clear although they admit the fact, but some of the women, who seemed to be fed up by the misbehavour of their husbands, said ironically that it is far better to have a daughter than a son who will be a liability like his father.

A noteworthy observation was that, abortion was also common among the women and even young unmarried girls had undergone secret abortion. The ANM plays an important role in all this set up. Some of the ANMs who conduct deliveries, are also supposed to be expert in abortions. Some serious cases of maternal or infant mortality were also reported but this did not seem to be a very serious problem in these regions.

Regarding family planning measures like use of contraceptive, operations or pills, it is the women who take the initiative. These are supplied by the ANM from the health centres but men feel ashamed to buy them from the bazaar.

Pregnancy is supposed to be an auspicious period especially in tribes and the woman is sheltered from evil spirits. She is given proper diet if the financial means permit. The women do go to the centres for proper check up during pregnancy. But most of the respondents have said that the child delivery is performed at home by ANM or by village nurse called Dai or Sayani (old experienced woman), with the help of a sterilized knife. Asked whether it has given rise to problems like septic or excessive bleeding, they pointed out that it happens sometimes but not often, and then the woman is taken to a hospital.

Most of the mothers are given normal diet after delivery and period of rest after delivery is also not very long. Generally they start doing household work after two weeks, the elderly women take care of the newly born child. Women who live in nuclear families, when they go to work out of home, they take their infant with them even after the fifteen days of child birth. Asked whether any religious ceremony is performed, they told that the woman is supposed to be polluted for fifteen days and she is not allowed to enter the kitchen or any household work till Puja is performed on the 11th day. But the woman is sent to work in the fields even after 3 days of delivery. There are certain taboos on some foods which are forbidden for her. The prescribed rest period for the mother is of 40 days but it is not in practice in hills. Most of the mothers breast feed their children, that also affect their health because they do not take extra nutrition. They get some tonics from the health centres but it is reported by ANM that women don't take them regularly. Pre-mature births sometimes create problem for the women.

Cultural Beliefs and Religious Practices

In chapter VI, specific convictions and beliefs associated with the health, sickness, disease, pregnancy, child birth and care of mother and child had been discussed. From the collected data and by observation, it came to notice that elderly women believe in the influence of evil spirits and protection of mother child from them, the young women do not seem to be very serious about them and generally they think that child birth and problems of disease and poor health etc., all are related either on circumstances or on the fate of person. Hakims or Ojhas are not so very common in these regions, which shows that women are considerably aware of the new influences. However, the belief in the local gods and goddess is still very strong in this area and there are some living example where a sick woman (person) is cured of the disease by a mere touch of a person possessed by spirit.

Medical and Health Care Delivery System

In chapter VII, the available health care facilities in the studied areas have been assessed according to the collected data, field survey and interviews by the project director herself. Regarding the Medical and Health Care Delivery System as planned by the government, the situation is not very encouraging. Most of the women fail to use these facilities because of the location and approach of the health centres. More than 20 to 30 villages are attached to one centre. The researcher had visited a few of them. Some centres had a doctor, a pharmacist, ANM, and menial staff. There was a separate room for the check up and delivery room in maternity centres also. An MBBS doctor was also employed. But the patients using these facilities were mostly from the nearby villages. The problems for the villagers of deep remote areas is the difficulty of transportation as most of them have to walk on foot.

In many villages, there are only sub centres and not PHCs, there is no doctor attached with, only ANM and her mate assistant were whole-sole incharge who are available only upto 2 PM. Many times she has to visit villages under her, at that time the centre used to remained closed. There was acute shortage of medicines. Only iron and vitamin tablets and some devices for family planning were available in small quantity.

However, the ANM or the midwife seemed to be an important person in the lives of women. But the ANM were also more interested in making the money. Those belonging to the Urban region did not want to stay in the villages and the women complained that ANM hardly visits their village for months. The researcher cross checked their compliant. The ANM admitted that it was correct as she had to go many times to attend meetings at City Community Health Centres. She also told that she was more interested in going to visit in and near her home village and it was not possible to visit so many villages. The researcher did not find any female doctor in the areas. The role of the doctor is played by ANM only. In serious cases the patient is taken to the civil hospital.

The Primary Health Centres have problems of their own. They do not get the medicines in sufficient amount; there is no Vehicle (Ambulance) of their own, to pick up the patients in emergency. The doctor (MBBS) comes once or twice a week. Women have generally complained of lack of sympathy, rude behaviour and careless attitude of the employees. On the whole, the picture of the Primary Health Centres and their employees is not very encouraging. There were some private doctors who have settled there, married the hilly girls and they are doing a better job as they have become part and parcel of that area. Similarly, some ANM, who have permanently settled in that region, were doing better work.

In some areas, specifically in tribal hilly areas, a few Missionary Health Centres and some NGOs have taken the upper hand. Many uneducated and less educated respondents were thought them the true government hospitals. They were appreciating their behaviour and work. Some of these are very much popular such as **Lehman Hospital** in Herbertpur (Dehradun Distt.) and **SAMTA** in Bhimawala, Vikasnagar.

A few case studies have been presented of these NGOs and Missionary Institutions on the basis of intensive interviews with the project director, in Appendix 1.

A few NGOs organize camps, workshops and lectures programmes for the adolescents to make aware them about sex-education, dangers of rape and too-early marriages etc., such as **Pahel** in Kolhupani (Dehradun Distt.).

Regarding the situation of medical facilities, though both the hilly regions (Kumoun and Garhwal) of Uttaranchal Pradesh was dismal and insufficient for the needs of people, but Kumoun is poorer comparatively to Garhwal. Dehradun, being the Capital of the State, and being the nearer to the urban-culture, has greater advantage in this matter and women of this region were more health-conscious.

Pattern of Social Relationships and Social Support System

Chapter VIII, is devoted to identify the pattern of social relationships and social support from relatives and neighbours at the time of illness, disease, child birth or any other calamity. For rural and tribal communities, living in isolated and remote hilly areas, which are deprived from modern health care facilities, the social support from kith and kin and neighbours is very much valuable and precious at the time of crisis. Even in modern medical science, it is admitted that strong emotional ties and warmth in family and social relations have very significant role in the healing and treatment of diseases.

The people world over, wondered, how in India, inspite of poverty, deprivation and backwardness, people have enjoyed life with celebrations in joint families. The various festivals and cultural events, hold the people together and perhaps make them resistant to many health problems.

It was observed in the present study, that inspite of many types of health problems, none of the women has complained of the social problems or thought of going out of that region and settling anywhere else. They are emotionally bound with their land, their surrounding and their cultural past. They are happy and satisfied with the life they are leading. Nearly all of them have good and supportive relations with their relatives and neighbours.

They stand by each other in times of illness or emergency, and even help them financially also. Although the people of these regions are also divided on the basis of caste, but as far as social relations and support are concerned, they come for help. During intensive survey, it was observed in village that there was no water for 3 days in village and the Sarpanch of the village himself called for the Tanker, he waited three to four hours on road with the villagers, (who were from the low castes) to make available water for them. There was no environment of hatred or enmity. On the whole, the peaceful social homogeneity of the region has a positive influence on their health due to strong social support system.

To sum up the main findings of the study it may be said that due to culturally sanctioned secondary status of women in family and society, triple burden of social roles i.e. reproductive, domestic chores and labour in production for earning money – coupled with hardships of hilly geographical situation of the region, most of the women of the rural and tribal areas of Uttaranchal Pradesh were seemed more old than their actual age. Their pale and wrinkled faces, their weak and frail phisique and bent-backs, all these symptoms, tell the story of ill-health, poor economic condition, under nourishment, inadequate quality of medical and health care during illness, time of pregnancy and child-birth and overburdened labour, of women living in the hilly regions.

But it is noteworthy here, that through intensive field survey and interviews with the Project Director, one trend came as a surprise that women's chances for better health care and nutrition improve, as they pass the reproductive age and achieve the social status of 'mother-in-law'.

As far as the government health care delivery system, in the studied area, is concerned, it was apparent from the interpretation of data in chapter VII regarding the availability of medical facilities, it was observed, that only 58.83% respondents informed that there are some kind of medical facilities available in or nearby their villages (government and private both), but the distance from their residence was one to three kilometers. As much as 41.17% have answered that in their villages no such government centres or government medical facilities are available nearby their villages and they have to go in Cities or 'Kasbas' for treatment. However 10.78% have told that to avail the government medical facilities they have to travel more than six kilometers which is many times becomes impossible in the case of emergency.

As far as the question of Primary Health Centres (PHC) and Sub-Centres is concerned, only 28.84% have admitted that these centres are in functioning condition in their areas but the distance from their residence is one to three kilometres.

The frequency of visits of personnels of PHC or MHC such as Doctor or ANM, it was reported by the respondents that mostly these visits are once in a month and rarely once in a week in their villages. The kind of facilities available in the PHCs or MHCs are also not upto the mark, most of the centres have shortage of ambulance, oxygen cylinder, pathology lab, operation equipment or even costly medicines, injection and dressing materials. Only iron and vitamin tablets, cough syrups or pain-killers are available there, immunization facilities for children such as BCG or Polio drops are available at PHC to some extent. However family planning devices such as pills and other contraceptives are always available to touch the government targets. MBBS doctors in Primary Health Centres are in a very few numbers so most of the centres are running by Pharmacists and Maternity centres and sub-centres by ANMs. The reason may be that Indian physicians, "educated" in the logic of Private Health Care, did not dare to go up the hills to attend the need of population in the panorama of exclusion, precarious life conditions and difficult access.

The complaints of rude behaviour of medical personnels of government centres were also common among the villagers, perhaps the reason is over-burden of work. During field survey of PHC and MHC, it came to notice that as many as twenty, thirty to forty and sometimes number goes up to sixty villages are attached with one centre and there is always shortage of staff.

Regarding the utilization of medical facilities by the respondents, most of them reported that, although they go to these centres despite the long distance, because they cannot afford the expenses of private doctors or nursing homes, but they were not satisfied at all with the services of PHCs and MHCs, and about 34.83% respondents told that they never went to either PHC or government dispensaries. The reason for not going were several, such as lack of confidence on doctors, carelessness in treatment, rude behaviour of personnels, absence of doctors every time, shortage of medicines in the stock, too much long distance and lack of transportation facilities etc. Although these respondents were not economically well off and they had to manage money anyhow for treatment. But they were very much fed-up with these centres and they thought it was wastage of time and energy going there.

The only bright side of the social life of the people living in remote hilly areas, is that, despite the poverty and deprivation of modern facilities of life, these villagers belong to a strong social support system, due to integrated inter-relationship and warm emotional ties, among the members within the communities. They stand by each other in times of illness, child-birth or any other emergency and even they help each other financially also.

Part II

Examining the Hypotheses

After the analysis of main findings of the study, it will be pertinent to examine the hypotheses of the study on the basis of information collected through schedules, intensive interviews and observations.

The study hypothesized that health seeking behaviour differs from culture to culture. No doubt the health related norms, rules and beliefs regarding illness and treatment of any group or community are intimately related to its cultural traditions to some extent. As the present study shows that there prevail some restrictions about intake of food items, behavioural patterns and taboos regarding pregnancy, after child birth and during monthly periods even for unmarried girls. But these restrictions are not so specific as nearly all rural societies follow these taboos even in some orthodox urban families too, these things are common and followed even today.

During informal chat with a group of women, it came to notice that there exist a strong belief that some persons possess the super-power from good sprits for healing the incurable diseases, and the sick people were cured by a mere touch of such persons. They had described some experiences which confirm their beliefs in this regard.

But in general, women were considerably aware of modern-rational influences and there seemed no significant cultural differences in day-to-day routine and precautions regarding healthcare in these hilly regions.

The study also hypothesized that in traditions bound society, people ignore modern health services. The study did not show such trend. But in contrast the respondents had the preference for modern medical system and they were very much depressed because of the shortage of P.H.C., M.H.C. and modern health care facilities in government dispensaries for treatment in their villages. Although, generally women were careless for themselves to take treatment at once in the initial stage of illness, from allopathic doctor, but for their children, they were very much anxious to take them to allopathic doctors or to the city hospitals at once if their economic condition permit them.

Buddhadeb Chaudhari also observed this trend in his study and opined that, "there are a number of studies which have shown that when both the facilities, namely, traditional and modern are available, even tribals often accept the modern system of treatment." (Chaudhari, 1994).

The preference for modern health care system may be for these reasons such as proper diagnosis of the disease, more chances of immediate relief, attraction and utility of modern health equipments, cleanliness and hygienic atmosphere of clinics or hospitals etc.; So despite the shortage of finances, villagers prefer the modern healthcare system especially in case of serious diseases.

Regarding the quality of medical treatment and health care, the most important factor in the present time, is the economic status and earning capacity of the person or household. To assess the role of economic factors, the study hypothesized that "the health status is related to the financial condition of the family i.e. better economic status would imply better women's healthcare."

For the assessment of this crucial factor, it was experienced by the researcher during the whole process of the study that the women of remote hilly and tribal regions were living in conditions, full of hardships and over burdened labour, deprived from even minor facilities of livelihood, health care, nutrition, rest or recreation, proper care during pregnancy and child-birth or at the time of illness or disease. The only reason of such miserable life was non but poverty and less earning of income despite of hard labour. Economic factor is that pivotal element which decides the opportunities of life in every aspect, may be either standard of living and social status in society or quality of food, nutrition, healthcare, quality of medical treatment, kind of work and labour, duration of rest or recreation, mode of social relationships and contacts and what not!

The study found the obvious impact of economic status and earning capacity of the families on the health status and conditions of respondents to large extent. Poverty clubbed with hardships of remote hilly geographical infrastructure and acute shortage of water, all these crucial factors created many health hazards in the life of the hilly women.

The study has also assumed that educated women are more health conscious than their less or uneducated counterparts. As the data regarding education has shown in the study that as many as 60% women were educated in between the primary to intermediate level, though the number of highly educated women was very tiny. But the study did not show that education has too-much significant role in health-matters in hilly regions. Health issue, in these hilly region was found very much complicated and multifactoral problem. Caste structure, economic status, climatic and geographical structure, acute shortage of water and fuel, poor level of the availability of medical and health care facilities, lazyness and drunkardness of the male members of the families – all these factors impose the triple burden on women of hilly regions. Whether less educated or more educated, the fate of all women in these hills is more or less the same miserable one, unless they are from rich families and at the same time from high caste groups.

Part III

Analysis and Suggestions

An Evaluative Analysis of the Current Health Policy of the Government

The findings of this study present a dismal and depressing picture of Indian Villages especially of the remote hilly and tribal villages of Uttaranchal Pradesh in health, hygiene, sanitation and medical care related issues which are the matter of serious concern for the nation.

The first citizen of the country, the president of the world's largest democracy, A.P.J. Abdul Kalam in his book 'India 2020 (1998)' has expressed his anxiety for the nation in these words, "after the six decades of independence, India needs such very basic essentials even today as 'to remove poverty of millions people; to provide health for all; to provide employment opportunities for all; ...., and to be self-reliant in national security and build-up capabilities to sustain and improve on all these in future." APJ Abdul Kalam (1998).

The analysis of health scenario of the studied villages vis a vis to the health scenario of the whole country, presents some serious paradoxes of the health policy of the government. Fifty five years ago, the leaders of the newly independent India, had promised to their country people, in the preamble of constitution, to establish a 'progressive socialistic pattern of society based on the principles of liberty, equality, fraternity and social justice' – a true incarnation of 'Democratic Welfare State'. In the directive principles of the constitution, the welfare of women, children, downtrodden and scheduled castes and tribes, was given the topmost priority, as its target of national planning. The issues, such as health, hygiene, sanitation and child-welfare and family planning, were set out as the important part of the health-policy of the government. No doubt that the intention, goals and policies of the newly independent nation's government regarding health problems of the masses, were appreciable.

In the recent years, the government has revived its national health policy and many crucial steps have been taken, such as in the year 1978, India has become a signatory member of the 'Alma Ata' declaration and committed to achieve 'Health for All' by the year 2000. After that, in the National Health Policy, the Indian government included schedule castes and scheduled tribes as priority groups. "The document of 'Health for All' has a need based approach and helping achieve the goal through universally accessible health care with a tolerable level of quality determined by the affordability of a community." (Godwin S.K. 2004). In 2002, "The National Health Policy has set out the goal of providing world-class medical care at a fraction of the cost incurred in the developed countries in India due to the availability of relatively cheaper but quality manpower, low priced drugs and other infrastructure. The slogan has been 'First World Treatment at Third World Prices'." Gupta (2004).

No doubt, there is flooded increase in corporatized health institutions and Apollo Hospitals in the country, since last two decades. "And the fancy buildings, plush surrounding and hi-tech-equipments of these Apollo Hospital groups fascinate the rich 'consumer's' perception for availing quality medical services." Baru (2002).

The capacity of modern-medical system in India, to provide high-quality medical care on unprecedented scale on comparatively one-fourth or one-fifth cost (four or five times cheaper) to UK or US, is a major achievement on the part of Indian Medical System. This tremendous progress, in the health and medical field, has risen the new hopes in Indian politicians and ministers to enrich the country's foreign-exchange fund. They are thinking the 'Health and Medical Matter' as a profitable industry and name it 'Medical Tourism'.

Renuka Chaudhary, the union minister of state for tourism feels that "health tourism can emerge as a foreign exchange earner for the country given its advantages." (The Hindu, Chennai, June 8, 2004). The former finance minister Jaswant Singh, "in his last year budget, called for India to become a 'Global Health Destination'." (The Financial Times, July 2, 2003).

The urge for promoting medical tourism, received further impetus from the prime-minister's council for trade and industry, led by Kumarmanglam Birla and Mukesh Ambani, which identified it as a potential 'Sunshine Industry'. The National Health Policy 2002, also unambiguously legitimate the concept, when it reads "to capitalize on the comparative cost advantage enjoyed by domestic health facilities in the secondary and tertiary sector, the policy will encourage the supply of services to patients of foreign origin, on payment in foreign exchange will be treated as 'deemed exports' and will be made eligible for all fiscal incentives extended to export earnings." (as quoted in Gupta, 2004) "Due to the attraction of foreign exchange and the concern for economic growth, the government is willing to offer fiscal and policy incentives to such ventures and thus India is emerging as a major medical tourism market player." (Godwin S.K., E.P.W. Sept 4, 2004).

What may be the possible implications of promoting medical tourism, through corporate medical institutions, on the concept of public health, cost of health care and equity of the national health system, the national target of 'health for all' etc., one can easily estimate the dangers and crisis for the majority of Indian masses. For not only the rural masses, but for even average urban Indian patient, the cost of treatment in a five-star hospital, is mere a dream, even for upper-middle class people, it is beyond reach, affordable only to some richest-classes. "The huge difference in the cost of treatment between foreign hospitals and Indian corporate hospitals is also a major pull factor for the so-called external 'brain-drain' in which developed countries are the major beneficiaries, because they have higher priced currency than the third world countries." (Godwin, 2003). The same deviance is true within India as well. "The urban-centric corporate hospitals are drawing away the best-qualified personnels from the public sector. This absorption by private corporates imposes huge costs on the public health services by deteriorating, the quality of public health services." (Godwin, S.K., Sep. 4, E.P.W. 2004).

How amazing the concept of 'Medical Tourism' for a country, where about 40 percent people of its total population are living in acute miserable conditions of life i.e. below the poverty line, even today. And another 20 to 30 percent people are living only upto subsistence level, despite hard physical labour. A society where "diseases arising from poverty, ignorance, malnutrition, bad sanitation, lack of drinking water, inadequate housing and low levels of humanity, are still rampant." (Sachidanand, 1994). A nation, where substantial proportion of population is unable to receive even minimally adequate medical care and due to shortage of money, people waiting for treatment in never-ending long queues in front of government dispensaries or hospitals. In such a country, talking about the 'Medical Tourism' is nothing but a sheer injustice to the already deprived and distressed masses of the country.

The nation-wide data about the Public-Health Care System, tells this major paradox of modern medical system in India. According to a report of United Nations Development Programme, the expenditure on health of Indian government is lowest in the world. India spends only 0.9% from its GDP on the health of its people, it means $ 4, per head in a year. P. Sainath stated "There is very little, that is public, left in the sphere of health-care. Since Public spending is mere 0.9 percent of GDP in India, down there with the worst level." (P. Sainath, the Hindu, Jan. 4, 2006). The implications of this policy are very harmful for poor masses. U.N. Human Development Report, 2005 puts it "some of India's southern cities may be in the midst of a technology boom, but one, in every 11, Indian children dies in the first five years of life, for want of low-technology, low-costs interventions." (The Hindu, Jan. 4, 2006). It is observed through a survey by 'The Hindu' that, "medical care is now the second most common cause of rural family debt. The reason is obvious that people do not rely upon the very low-grade health care services rendered by public health care institutions."

On the other hand, many of India's giant corporate hospitals got millions of rupees in public subsidies. Dr. K.N. Nagraj of the Madras Institute of Development Studies stated that, "The Indian Health Sector is among the most privatized in the world .....our health expenditure data show that clearly. Very few nations have lower public health spending (as a share of GDP) than our own. On the other hand, may be just 12 developing nations exist where private spedning on health (as a share of GDP) is more than India." (K.N. Nagraj, The Hindu, Jan. 4, 2006). "The share of private corporates spending on health is only just 3 percent. The rest of the more than Rs. 1000,000 crores, that is spent on health, comes from ordinary households. It is, what the Indian people pull out of their own torn pockets. And their spending is growing at about 14 percent a year....... The damage has much to do with the gutting basic public services. It has a lot to do with rising inequality." (P. Sainath, The Hindu, Jan. 4, 2006) "The poor cannot hope for even the bare minimums now. Not in the age of market fundamentalism." (Ibid).

The mindless privatization of health sector has created serious scarcity of health-care facilities for the poor masses. In the public health department, India has 7.4 Lakh nurses, 3.5 Lakh chemists, 1500 hospitals, 8,70,000 beds only, which means

94 beds on 1,00,000 people, which is less than International Standard of minimum 333 beds. There is three-tier system in rural areas. In the towns and villages, there are 23,000 Primary Health Centres (PHC), 13,700 sub-centres and 3,000 Community Health Centres. Among these, 10 percent PHCs, which are in secluded remote villages, have no doctors. In the matter of Primary Health Care, India stands too much below of International standards. According to an estimate, India has only 43 doctors on 1,30,000 people. "It means government hospitals at present require atleast 40,000 more doctors and enormous para-medicals." (Asha Krishna Kumar, Frontline, Dec. 4, 2004).

In this perspective one can imagine the health condition of Indian people, particularly the condition of women's health who are the least persons to receive health care facilities and treatment during illness and disease and even during pregnancy and child birth. "Maternal health is a serious problem in India. It is estimated that nearly 1,36,000 women die each year due to causes related to pregnancy, child birth and abortion." (The Hindu, Dec. 28, 2005). "India has an estimated maternal mortality ratio (MMR) of 540 deaths per 1,00,000 live births, which means one woman dying every five minutes." (The Hindu, 28th Dec., 2005). The constitution of India guarantees the right to equality and the right to life including the right to health. Despite this, India has the highest MMR in South Asia. Being the most populous country of the world, India's 0.9% expenditure on health sector shows, acute imbalance of allocation of its total GDP on various developmental schemes. Dr. Vaidyanathan from Jawahar Lal National University of Social Medicine and Community Health Centre stated that, "In 1947, Government of India had decided to spend minimum 12% on health from its GDP, but even in its best days, government could not touch this figure." (Dr. Vaidyanathan, Frontline, Dec. 4, 2004).

The small amount of expenditure on health sector by the Indian Government, as mentioned above (only 0.9%) has further deteriorated the public health care system which was already in its worst possible condition as depicted in recent 'Comments' by renowned writer and journalist Mrinal Pandey in her article "जनस्वास्थ्य सुविधाओं की शवसाधना" in a prestigious news paper "हिन्दुस्तान" Dated Jan. 15, 2006. The article is based on the reports of several surveys done by public interest agencies. The relevant lines of the article are presented here as such .... "हमारी राष्ट्रीय उत्पाद दर भले ही 8 प्रतिशत का आंकड़ा छू रही है, लेकिन जनस्वास्थ्य सूचकांक शर्मनाक हैं। 90 प्रतिशत स्त्रियाँ तथा बच्चियाँ चिन्ताजनक रक्ताल्पता की शिकार हैं, 70 प्रतिशत किसी न किसी प्रजनन तन्त्र सम्बन्धी रोग को भोग चुकी हैं या उसकी गिरफ्त में हैं, टायफायड, हैपेटाइटिस, मलेरिया और कालाजार जैसे रोग महामारी बन कर फैल रहे हैं।..................सरकारी अस्पतालों में न पर्याप्त डाक्टर बचे हैं, न संसाधन, न ही चिकित्सा उपकरण।..................जब तक हमारा सार्वजनिक स्वास्थ्य तन्त्र हमारे करोड़ों जरूरतमन्द लोगों को निराश खाली हाथ लौटाएगा, जब तक गांव में जाकर प्राथमिक स्वास्थ्य केन्द्रों में कार्य करने वाली नर्सों का जीवन असुरक्षित रहेगा, अवैध दवाओं की फैक्ट्रियाँ, अवैध कारखानों से नकली दवाओं के अंबार लगाती रहेंगी, तब तक अप्रशिक्षित और प्रायः हानिकारक नीम हकीमी स्वास्थ्य – उपचारों की जड़ें नष्ट नहीं होंगी।"

"..................हमारी दलगत (प्रायः जाति, धर्म के सांचों में गढ़ी गई) राजनीति ने भी बेवकूफी भरे या काईयाँ हस्तक्षेप द्वारा सार्वजनिक क्षेत्र की जनस्वास्थ्य सुविधाओं से लगातार खिलवाड किया है। संसाधन हों न हों, अपने चुनाव क्षेत्र में जबरन अस्पताल या डिस्पेन्सरी खुलवाना, प्राथमिक स्वास्थ्य केन्द्र कर्मियों से जब–तब स्वास्थ्य मेले आयोजित कराके, उनको खुद चुनावी मंच की तरह इस्तेमाल करना, बड़े सरकारी अस्पतालों से हर तरह की सुविधा खुद घर बैठे मंगवाना और डाक्टरों की नियुक्ति तथा प्रमोशन में धांधली, इन हथकंडों ने हमारी सरकारी चिकित्सा और शिक्षण संस्थानों का कबाड़ा कर ड़ाला है।" Pandey (2006).

Having briefly discussed the various aspects of the health scenario of the country, with particular reference to Rural and Tribal villages of Uttaranchal Pradesh, the researcher humbly means to say that the Health Care System of our country requires renewal, repair and reconstruction. For this purpose, following suggestions may be useful.

Recommendations and Suggestions

1. To make health–care system pro-poor, pro-rural and pro-underprivileged classes of the country, a revolutionary change in national health policy is required, which will mean, the basic transformation in the strategy of health related planning and programmes. To achieve the goal of 'Health for All by 2000', the first and foremost condition is to change the direction of health policy towards public interest instead of to make it the tool of profit earning industry for the corporate world. For this purpose the major proportion of the health-expenditure should be chanalized towards rural and tribal health schemes. Only, a strong political will and firm national commitment at the highest ministerial level can serve the purpose.

2. Health matter is a complex phenomenon, which involves so many factors in it, especially in hilly rural areas. So health policies must be integrated into programmes of economic, social and community development for these areas. Joint schemes with such sectors as agriculture with other opportunities of employment and livelihood, education, means of transportation and communication in remote hilly areas, health and sanitation awareness based community programmes with adequate understanding of socio-cultural background of hilly rural groups, especially of tribal groups must be taken as the part of health policy.

3. Mostly in hilly regions of Uttaranchal Pradesh, the economy of the poor households is forest based. Women

of these households make provision for basic necessities like food, fuel, fodder for their cattle, and tissues of plants for making clothes etc. There should be relaxation in the forest policy of the government for the entry of hilly people in jungles and their traditional forest rights should be restored.

4. Acute shortage of safe drinking water is the major problem of hilly region. Although it is countrywide problem as observed by I.K.Gujral (Former Prime minister of India) "I see before me the bottled water kept for the dignitaries on the dais. It reminds me of three classes of Indians; one who can afford bottled water, other who manage to get some water in their taps, or in nearby tap or a pump, irrespective of its quality; the third set of Indians are those, for whom drinking water is a daily problem and who will be ready to drink any polluted water." "For such a situation to persist after fifty fives years of independence was a national shame", he added. (An address by I.K.Gujral in science Congress at Hydrabad in, 1998).

   In hilly regions of Uttaranchal Pradesh, the problem is of third category in regard of drinking water. Solution of this problem should be given on priority basis in the health care system of the government. Programmes like watershed development should continue but not in ritualistic way but in proper, careful initiative of villages and government.

5. According to the latest National Family Health survey, half of all Indian children are undernourished and half of all adult women suffer from anemia. Vaccination is looked at as a solution instead of improving nutrition, safe drinking water and sanitation, which will automatically raise resistance levels to diseases. The focus on vaccines has meant that routine health services and

basic health facilities have suffered. There should be combine campaign to the treatment in this regard.

6. Government should have to make genuine attempt to provide medical health care to the masses, as government is abdicating its responsibility to the private agencies, is not correct policy. Government should make direct interference in health policy and stop it to convert it to commercial product. In the medical Colleges passed students should have compulsory services in the villages.

7. Schemes like 'National Cooked Nutritious Mid Day Meal Scheme' and integrated child development services (ICDs) 'Anganwadi' in every village should be functional and supervised properly. It should be ensured full coverage for all the villages of the hilly and Tribal areas.

8. Primary Health Care Centres are the key source and an important constituent of the government health care system in the villages. As apparent from the countrywide data especially in the remote hilly areas, these basic institutions are in very few number in the comparison to the needs of the people. So immediate steps should be taken to increase the number of primary health centres and sub centres with full facilities in the remote areas all over the country.

9. As data regarding the health care facilities reveals that everywhere, there is shortage of staff in already existing PHCs in the villages, as much as 38 percent of all Public Health Centers (PHC) have the acute shortage of staff. Health family surveys conducted by the International Institute of Population Sciences (Mumbai) show that only 69 percent of PHCs have at least one bed and 20 percent have a telephone. There is immediate requirement of new recruitment in post of doctors and Para medicos.

10. The government needs to re-examine the current drug pricing policy. The numbers of drugs that are under price control have come down from 347 in the 1979 Drug Price Control Order to the current 74. The National Pharmaceutical Policy for 2002 suggests that this be further reduced to 34. But this should be revised and there should be price control over life saving drugs to make available for the poor and lower middle classes.

These, and several other necessary measures may lead the Indian health care system towards the direction of 'Democratization'.

Appendix - I

Case Studies

Introduction

In Appendix I, a few case-studies have been presented on the basis of intensive field survey and personal interviews, with several Primary Health Centres, Sub-Centres, Doctors, ANMs, NGOs and influential social workers of the studied area by the Project Director herself.

The purpose of presenting the case studies, adjoined with the report, is to bring into light those salient but hidden 'atoms' and 'molecules' related to every aspect of health-scenario, which were not possible to produce through the findings, based on the routine interview-schedules, filled by the investigators. Case studies are the outcome of informal dialogues, experiences and impressions on Project Director with the respondents, and health-related personnels and institutions, during field survey. This effort may serve the purpose to make the study more informative, objective and close to reality.

All the twelve case studies, represent their peculiar nature and role, whether Christian Missionary Hospital, NGOs, Doctors or ANMs, Social Workers, Primary Health Centres, village of Jaunsar Bawar or a common woman like Kaushalya Devi, everyone is playing a role, big or small, in the health scenario of their particular society. For making better understanding of general health scenario of the country, these individuals or institutions become a key point.

Note : For the sake of secrecy, names of the individuals have been changed.

Case Study I

Primary Health Center and Maternity Health Centre Raipur Block (District Dehradun)

Researcher has visited a few Primary Health Centres, one of them is PHC in Raipur Block, Dehradun District. It was well built building of seven rooms, one was for doctor, one for Pharmacist, one for office purpose and other employees, another two rooms with two beds each for patients, and one dressing room. In this PHC total 14 persons are employed. One male and one female doctor, one pharmacist, three health superintendents, two health visitors, one supervisor, one ANM and her assistant mid-wife (Dai) and three peons (4th class employees).

Almost, people of fifty villages are attached with this PHC. Every type of patient visits there. Especially patients of stomach related problems, general weakness, child-problem, immunization, accidents and other injuries come here. Researcher accompanied with an influential social worker and her two companions, reached at the centre at 1 O'clock. Till this time doctor had left his cabin. But at that time so many patients were there whom pharmacist was providing medicines and consultancy. Closing time of PHC was 2 O'clock. There was one patient, who was admitted for one day in the PHC.

Pharmacist after attending the patients, talked to Researcher. Researcher had discussed many issues such as, about type of patients, their attitude towards treatment and health care, facilities available etc. Pharmacist revealed that due to conveyance problem, patients of remote villages usually default in taking proper treatment. So, many women sent their husbands or sons after detailing them about problems. This becomes tedious job for doctor to give correct medicine. Almost

150-200 patients regularly come in PHC for consultation. One doctor is not enough for it. Patients have to wait for a long. Due to over burden of work, doctor cannot visit the villages. In emergency cases, there is no facility like oxygen cylinder, ambulance. Because of lack of proper transportation, patients suffer a lot.

The Maternity Health Center has two rooms, one as office room for ANM, another for patients like dressing room. ANM sees patients for two times, 11.00 to 2.00 p.m. in the morning and at evening 5.00 to 7.00 pm. According to her, patients of leocoria and loop-related problems, weakness before and after pregnancies come usually. She only gives iron and vitamins and contraceptives like Mala-D, Condoms etc. ANM told Researcher that a few women, come at the time of some serious delivery case, to seek doctor's help, otherwise most the deliveries are done by ANM and mid wife at the patient's homes. ANM and dai both have over-burden of work. At the time of complication, patient's family rush to Dehradoon. Other poor patients come at center but due to insufficient transportation facilities and awareness, mother and child both caught in the risk of life. ANM also cannot visit in the prescribed villages regularly. Mostly patients come at the centre, every time there exists scarcity of medicine at the centre, even sending so many reminders is usual practice. Remote and scattered villages, poverty, lack of staff and medicine, no ambulance and over burden task, create dismal picture of health care system in remote area of Uttaranchal Pradesh's Rajdhani.

Case Study II

Dr. Mrs. Sharma (A Gynecologist in Government Hospital)

At about 2 to three kilometers of distance from Almora, there is a Government Hospital known as Base Hospital in Katyari village in Almora District. The Project Director visited this Hospital, surveyed its situation and working. In this process, she came into contact with a Gynecologist, who was very much considerate and concerned with the health problems of hilly women, especially with their reproductive health. The project director made request her to share her experiences about the health condition of women of this region. The substance of this conversation is mentioned as follows.

In the hilly terrain where traveling hazards are most serious, the most deaths occur among women during pregnancies, Dr. Sharma said with grief on her face. Pregnancy is blatantly seen as a very trivial phenomenon in a society where women's health is the least preferred thing; it becomes more glaring act when it should be given a serious thought. Women have to deal with mundane chores like fetching water to steep heights, and collecting wood from the forests, remain their tasks as per their daily schedule, even during pregnancy, apart from household work, which they have to deal with. Very little medical aid is available to them and whatever is there, is in the hands of unscientific and untrained midwives and elderly women which often make a mess of this situation. Untimely and improper medical aid is the cause of death of most women during this time. Even when there is serious complication, time taken to the reach a hospital, is so due to hilly region and no transport, that the women dies on the way. Even when they reach hospital after such huge delays, they get uterus and ovary related complications, which becomes a cause for future health problems.

Dr. Sharma had told about a delivery case of a woman from a well to do family where, there was no financial problem, the time taken to reach the hospital was 5 hours due to hilly region and long distance. After reaching the hospital after such a long journey, to save the life of women was a tedious job. After five hours long operation, the newborn child had the ill fate of death. Such cases are large in number in this region.

Dr. Sharma is very sensitive to the problems of this region. She feels an urge to do something to the problems of women apart from her routine duties, at the base hospital. She travels to the remote areas at this hilly region and gives information on pregnancy related problems to the women of this region. She has carved out her task, her goals are clear and she wants full co-operation from the govt as well. She wants midwives in villages to be properly trained scientifically, so that every village can have proper medical care, and some medicines, so that lives of women may be saved.

Case Study III

Dr. Naren (A Young Private Practitioner)

Dr. Naren is from Calcutta, after completing his BAMS in a very young age, came to Dehradun to take a chance for employment. In the very starting, he was willing to do some of social work through his service. He started his practice in a small village 'Paunda', Sahaspur Block, District Dehradun. He came just for trial. New language, new environment, and new culture, everything tried to force him to go back. He suffered with dual feeling, conscious is saying to continue, nostalgia calling at coast of west Bengal. In these circumstances he met a primary school teacher as his patient, meeting converted in to long life friendship. Dr. Naren has a quality to listen others; to take interest in small details of his patients. People of nearby villages mostly women and children come to him as his patients. His popularity grew but he was intimate only with the family of primary school teacher. The primary teacher and other villagers thought, that there is possibility of going back of Doctor without family life. To make him stay at paunda, old friend teacher proposed him to marry in that village with his daughter due to his gentle behaviour. Because of doctor's nature and service, primary school teacher broke all the bars of caste and region, married his daughter to the doctor. Now it took 14 years Dr. Naren is one of the part of this area.

When he was consulted about type of patients, he answered that most of the women come for Luocoria, anemia, T.B., backache problem, fertility etc. Dr. Naren is concerned about the miseries, poverty, mal-nutrition and hard life of hilly women. He only takes very nominal fees 10 rupees. Sometimes he does not take fees from poor people and provide medicine free, which he gets as a sample medicine. Dr. Naren's concern, his vision and simplicity give a way, which type of doctors villager's need.

Case Study IV

An A.N.M. (In a Primary Health Centre, Almora Distt.)

ANM's are appointed by the Health Department in every Primary Health Centre, Sub Centre and Maternity Health Centre in villages. They are properly trained personnels in Para-medical profession. They are meant to provide expert and scientific medical aid to pregnancy related problems of the women of that region. But ANM's are lowly paid and heavily work loaded. Many times low skilled women came into this professions, which create the risk for women's health, they work upon. But many women who get proper skills in their job do not hesitate to make commercial use of their skill, and to over look their duty in remote villages. They make profit in spending their duty time in the cities to perform the delivery cases and misuse their expertise and government job for profit motive.

During survey of a Community Health Centre in Almora the researcher was informed about the story of one such ANM. The people told researcher that rumours about such ANM has come to light in the health camp, which was organized by the Health Department. Various Doctors and other ANM's also knew about this particular ANM. They also complained that instead of staying on duty in her village, where she is posted, she stays in the city, and in her place of work, she contracted with a compounder who is posted in that P.H.C. For this purpose, she paid some commission to that compounder. Although when she was newly appointed, she worked well in her P.H.C. and she got popularity in the region. But after some time, when she became confident and popular, she started to spend her skill to make money out of it. She contracted also with other several midwives of this region and got cases through them and increased her profit. Women from well off families in cities and villages also call her for their problems, checkups and many times for delivery cases also. Due to compounder she goes in her own primary health center twice in a month or once in a week to mark her presence. These observations, forced to think that because of ANMs are paid small amount of salary and deprived from other facilities in the villages, they compensate their shortage of money with the commercial use of their skill and training. But the ultimate deprived sufferers are the women of the villages and not the ANMs.

This case study is the real picture of a common personnel who work in the Government Health Care System of the country to large extent.

Case Study V

An A.N.M. Madhu

(Sub-Health Centre, Village Paunda, District Dehradun)

Madhu now, almost forty-five years old Bengali woman, married with a Garhwali boy fifteen years ago. She took the training of ANM (auxiliary nurse midwife) as her keen interest in this profession. She is serving in Paunda Village, Sahaspur

Block, Dehradoon District since about twelve years. She has two children, one daughter and one son. Her husband is working a job in private institution. At present she is living in a three room rented residence where one room is used as dispensary for patients and small two rooms and kitchen for her. This is residence cum Sub Health Center. Main P.H.C. is situated in Premnagar (District Dehradun), four to five kilometers far away from Paunda village.

Madhu has established good informal relations with her patients. Approximately, women of fifteen villages come to her for consultancy, treatment of pregnancy related problems and vaccination of children. She herself not visited frequently in the villages, she only goes for delivery cases or some times for routine visit. Every Wednesday is celebrated as immunization day; on this occasion Aaganwadi workers also came to help Madhu in vaccination process and at the time of Pulse Polio day. About diseases of women, she told that most of the women of this area are suffering from Leocoria, anemia and backache. She provides Iron capsules, Calcium tablets and some other cheap tonics and cough syrups.

Madhu told that for family planning purpose, women always complain that neither their husbands use condoms nor they get operations. The women have to take initiative in this matter. Madhu, herself distributes contraceptives to rural women-folk. Although, she cannot do regular visits in all the villages, attached to her sub centre. But she is always available at the centre full time for women so they are satisfied with her. Madhu is popular, among the local women, they have faith in her.

When asked about the problems in running the center, she described many difficulties such as shortage of medicines, oxygen cylinder, blood provision, ambulance and qualified female doctor in emergency of serious cases. She has over burden of work but she is providing her services to the local people of that region, amid scarce means.

Case Study VI

Vandna

(An Influential Social Worker Sponsoring Several NGOs)

Kaparkhan and Kasar Devi are known to be a beautiful tourist spots of the hills of Kumaoun in Almora District. But beneath its scenic beauty, lies the story of tragic tales of the people of this region. Poverty, hard labour and lack of basic facilities of life, like – water, sanitation and health are the other faces of this region. Some people have the reason to make money out of every human tragedy and so has been done by an influential woman social worker Vandna. But let us understand Vandna first.

Vandna was born in an influential Bengali family, which lives in Almora for a long time. Her father was Bengali but mother was foreigner woman. Her parents had high-level connections in and out of the country both. The family was very rich and had so many lands and had the ownership of a big estate. Vandna was brought up in Kumaouny culture and language. She got higher education and got specialization in English language, but she speaks very good Kumaouny language also. She made good relationships with the people of her region. Being the native of hilly area, she had an understanding of miseries and poverty of the women of this hilly region.

To establish herself among the people she operated many health and job oriented schemes. The first effort of Vandna was to establish a hospital in Dina-pani near Kasar Devi, which was initially a primary health centre, having only a pharmacist there. But with her influence and acquaintances with the district authorities, she got the permission to expand that centre and acquired more land and converted it into a big hospital. Now the hospital has many high-class types of equipment, machines and high-class pathology lab and many qualified doctors. This hospital is famous for it's best treatment. Many girls from neighboring areas are getting employment here after receiving the training of nursing and midwifery. Due to this hospital, the people of this area now are getting better medical treatment but with spending a lot of money, while earlier, people used to get free medical aid from P.H.C.

The women are getting every kind of medical treatment, especially for pregnancy related problems and at the time of serious delivery cases, but they have to arrange money for this purpose.

Vandna has started a small-scale woolen industry to spin and weave shawls, carpets and woolen garments etc. For this purpose she has a direct contact and trade relations with 'Tibet', she employed many women form villages of Almora and she had grown the work on large scale in short time. Although poor women are getting money and employment but this was very less in comparison of their labour. In this way Vandna was making heavy profit by the exploitation of women's labour due to their accute need for job.

To harness the beauty of Kumoun hills, Vandna through her connections has pressurized the government to make the fifty kilometer of Binsar forest – a sanctuary and she also rendered her help to the government in doing so. To enjoy the beauty of Binsar forest, many tourist came to this place. To make the profit of this situation, she made a huge hotel in Kasar Devi Matt which itself is an attractive tourist destination. She has established herself as social worker and has established several N.G.O.s on the name of social work with aid of World Bank and it's several organizations. But due to her hidden profit-making interest, some people of that area have started to criticize her. The old generation of this region is very much dissatisfied and there is huge resentment in the areas of Kaparkhan, Kasar Devi, Sora and Tiladi etc. due to the huge arrival of foreigner tourists who are responsible in breaking the social fabric, and simplicity of this area.

Case Study VII

Kaushalya Devi

(A Resident of Village Kasar Devi Matt)

Kaushlya Devi, a sixty years old widow, with thin physique and wrinkled face, is the inhabitant of Village of Kasardevi Matt, District Almora. She was married in age of 16, became widow in age of 18. After her widowhood she lived only for two years in her in-law's house and then she came back to her parental house. Her parents died after few years. She had two younger brothers one is in Delhi, and another is in the village.

She lives with elder one. Her brother who is living in village is educated up to 10th standard. They have small holding of land. They took a plot on the roadside, constructed four rooms, one room converted in provisional store, keeping small essentials. This place matters for them, it comes on the way of two famous tourist spots, Kasar Devi and Binser. Mostly tourists want to stay on this route, Kaushalya's brother developed his two rooms in short stay home. This effort improved their economic condition. Kaushlya's brother is married, has two children. From 18 years up to this time neither Kaushalya, nor other members of her family, thought about her re-marriage. Her In-laws are in the same District, where she goes on special occasions. She does not get any financial help from them. At the home of her brother, she works whole day. She looks after children, fetch water and does another household works. Her brother's wife cooks meals both the time only. Researcher asked her daily routine and specifically about her health. She replied that she has always backache, joint-pain, but she does not mind it and does not take rest in the whole day. She takes rest at the time of heavy fever. She only one time became very seriously ill, that time, her younger brother called her in Delhi for the treatment, but after a little recovery, she came back to her mountains, as she was not feeling at ease there. Kaushalya claims herself healthy but Researcher observed at the time of interview, that she was weak and anemic and she was replying on every thing in a very pessimistic and detached manner as if she has no interest in life. Researcher asked her about food, she told that milk of Cow is for children, then for male members of the family, sometimes there is extra, she gives it to her sister-in-law. She takes tea only. In her daily food, she takes dal, rice and some vegetables, if available in kitchen garden. Though family of Kaushalya, is now well off, but they don't buy vegetables from market. Usually at the time of backache and headache, she takes tea with Tulsi or other herbal tea. Kaushlya keeps herself always busy even at the time of interview, she was grinding masala. In these two hours of interview she took 'bidi' twice just as a short break.

Case Study VIII

Kunna - Dakura (A Tribal Village) District Dehradun

It is the western part of 'Pachhuadoon', Uttaranchal Pradesh, confined between Yamuna and Tons (rivers) which forms the Jaunsar-Bawar. Kunna Dakura, a village distant about 5 to 6 km. from Chakrata, is distinct for its uniqueness. Jaunsar-Bawar area is known for its secret practices, relating religion and magic. Polyandry is still found in this area. It is a typical marriage institution, wherein a woman could have more than one husband simultaneously. This polyandrous institution is known here as Pandav-Vivah.

Project director, herself visited in this village through contact of a woman, who is working as a teacher in a Govt. School there. The Project Director, during her journey to the village, met on the way with the young girls and boys working in their narrow terraced fields at the season of harvesting. This was her first perception of this village. She talked to them in the fields, then they all accompanied her on the way to their village. This one of the blessed region of Himalaya where 'Mahasu Devta' reign, is very welcoming in nature. Devdar is the most important wood species of this area – and has been put to diverse structural uses. It has been extensively used for building houses and temples. All the houses of this village were neat and clean made by wood of devdar. These houses, its closets, almira, everything was unaffected by the attack of termites, looking as they were newly polished. In the houses of Kunna-Dakura, entrance or door is traditionally very small, that one has to bent. This was interpreted by villagers that one have to bow down to our culture and tradition before entering in our home.

This region is rich in natural vegetation. But agriculture is insufficient to earn livelihood by the people, they engage themselves in other vocations. Most of the male members of the village were out of the village – either in military services or any other manual labour. In agriculture, people have been growing coarse grains like maize, buckwheat, bathu, Rajma and ginger etc. which can withstand the dry and arid conditions. At the time of proper irrigation facility through the improvised channels, people also cultivate coarse variety of paddy. People of this village also keep cattle like goats and cows.

This village having fourteen to fifteen households, is culturally vibrant. As the project director was directed by teacher not to ask directly any question on polyandry, she followed. Project Director visited 6 to 8 households. In one of the family, where they visited a woman was married with three husbands (all were brothers) had four children. Another family had distinct example–elder brother married with two women but his two younger brothers will deemed as both the women's husbands. Primary school teacher told project director, that young generation especially 7th–8th class students of her school do not like this old age practice of polyandry and students told her, that in their turn, they will marry with single person.

At the first glance, village is not in bad condition. Women seemed to be healthy, slim and active. Elderly women were comparatively healthy as they have less burden to run the family. Drinking water is still a challenge here, women have to fetch water from long distance. Usually after converting a spring into a reservoir and provided by a tap, people use water.

In Kunna-Dakura village, there is no hospital or doctor, only one health visitor, who irregularly visit in their village. At the time of any physical problem, people come to Chakrata, where one PHC and other private doctors are available. Immunization and other minor problems are dealt by ANM who comes at the gap of one month. In a nearby village of Kunna-Dakura, there is one PHC but without doctor, only pharmacist deal with patients. No doctor wants to stay in this remote village. Usually due to climatic reasons doctors take transfer. Generally after November this region become locked with snow, roads blocked with ice upto February. There is one middle school I to VIII class. For further studies students go to Vikasnagar or Dehradun to continue their further studies.

In Kunna-Dakura, on the surface, women were looking healthy but actually they had problem of cervical, backache, tuberculosis. Due to their nature of hospitality and liveliness, villagers hide all their problems, at the time of telling about problems they only smile. Every family, visited by the researcher, had served 'Ladva' (a kind of sweet and salty papad) to the researcher as a symbol of hospitality.

They requested project director to stay at night, as that was their festival night, and the whole village together, had a singing and dancing programme at night in the moon light. In turn on the request of the teacher and project director, the young girls demonstrated a folk song with their traditional group dance in their sweet and melodious voice.

Case Study IX

Pehel (N.G.O.)

Adolescence is the most sensitive and delicate stage in journey of human life, in which nature has poured down spring of energies, creativity, curiosity, opportunities and unlimited possibilities with full heart. But this making period need a soft hand of a potter, otherwise risk of melting is ever-present. **'Pehel'** is an initiative in this direction. Project director met Pehel's area incharge Madam Kavita in their branch office in Kolupani, Sahaspur block, Dehradun district.

'Pehel', is working in the three districts, Dehradun, Udham Singh Nagar and Nainital, among young adolescents between the ages of 13 and 19 years are the focus of the initiative, which addresses their overall health and developmental needs. This was started in Dec. 2003 funded by Himalayan Institute Hospital Trust.

Young people between 10 to 24 years of age, constitute one third of the total population of India. Despite adolescent being a huge segment of population, policies and programmes in India, focused very little on adolescent group. According to 'Pehel', youth is period of acquiring new capacities and facing new challenges. It is a time of opportunity, but also of vulnerability to risk behaviour, which can have life long consequences, especially for health.

'Pehel's goal is to develop a shared understanding of the youth's needs within the state with respect to reproductive and sexual health, to develop advocacy forum based on broad issues pertaining to youth in the state of Uttaranchal. **'Pehel'** is the initial step in the process, 'a platform' for developing a shared understanding of the youth needs, within the state with respect to reproductive sexual health.

'Pehel' runs library for the awareness of adolescents. **'Pehel'** organizes group discussions, medical camps, poster exhibitions on the core issues of adolescents in the schools of field areas. Lack of knowledge, awareness, education on reproductive and sexual health issues, among young people, is cause of so many deviations in adolescents. So many problems related to menstruation are common among rural girls, knowledge related to puberty is lacking among adolescents, poor hygiene, physical abuse, prevalence of myths and misconceptions related to reproductive and sexual health, are common topics of discussion among the gathering organized by **'Pehel'**. Almost nine supervisors and so many trainees organize these programmes. They deal with psychological issues, adolescent nutrition, gender discrimination, stress among adolescents etc. in their workshops. **'Pehel'** does counseling among adolescents on various issues.

The best and most important period of life is childhood and if the right seeds are sown, then, one truly grows and develops — this is the work what **'Pehel'** is doing.

Case Study X

SMTA (N.G.O.)

'Society for Motivational Training and Action' is working in mountainous regions of District Dehradun and Uttar Kashi. It was in 1983 SWRL Tiloniya opened its branch at Chakrata, Dehradun District, but after three years, this unit

became independent unit. **Smta** believes in active community participatory development. Because of this belief, they give their major importance to awareness training to local social animators. These local social animators in turn give the required training to all the village communities, on a regular basis.

Smta is working in various fields of social activity, like primary education, community organization, through awareness building, promotion of community health, watershed development, non-conventional energy programme etc. At present SMTA is assisting the communities in two districts in Dehradun – Vikasnagar, Kalsi, Chakrata block and in Uttar Kashi - Naugaon and Purola.

Community Health, is an important area of the activity of **Smta**. It has its own community health centres, which provide health care, through their OPD. Time to time they held health camps and village health trainings. The school health programme is another important activity. These, one or two days camps, are held in the villages itself so that all mentors attend these camps. Usually topics on environmental sanitation, nutrition and personal hygiene, importance of universal immunization and reproductive health care education, (Pre natal and post natal health care), eye camp and lab-training camps and general health are organized by **Smta**. At the time of pulse polio programme **Smta**'s office become one of the centre in Vikasnagar.

Revival of traditional health care is one of the interesting programme of **Smta**. During its other projects, side by side **Smta** identified 18 traditional practitioners. After the training, the services of these traditional practitioners, have been increased. In this way multi-purpose work has been done. A number of local medicinal plants have been identified and they are under process of documentation. Eighteen nurseries have been established by these 'Vaidyas' in their respective villages so that they have an easy access to the medicinal plants in time of need.

Smta has introduced health education programme in all its “Apna School” which is run by its own volunteers. All the children of V standard and above, get health care inputs like personal hygiene, importance of immunization, reproductive health education and gastro-entices control through ORS.

Smta is funded by Indian and foreign agencies, which they get for the sake of charitable or religious propose. This N.G.O. is closely attached with Missionary services in Dehradun.

Case Study XI

Lehman – A Christian Missionary Hospital, Herbertpur (District Dehradun)

Lehman Missionary Hospital is situated in Herbertpur, Vikasnagar, Dehradun, on the foothills of Himalaya. This hospital was established by ‘Father Jeffery Lehman’ of U.K. in 1936 in this region. This ‘Christian Charitable Hospital’ is popular among local people as ‘Lemon Hospital’.

This hospital is playing major role in the life of majority of the hilly and tribal communities, who are struggling to make a living with degraded resource base. ‘Christian Missionary Hospital’ is part of ‘Emmaunal Missionary Trust.’ This hospital is well equipped, having hundred beds and all types of modern facilities.

This hospital is not charitable in conventional way. According to medical superintendent of the hospital, Dr. Sabu, “we do make profit to run this hospital.” Christian Missionary Hospital, does not take directly any fund from government or non-government organizations. But they get facility of low cost medicine and equipments. In this hospital 18 doctors among them – two Gynecologist, Paediatrics, Orthopaedic, psychologist, physiotherapist, surgeon etc. are available twenty four hours in the hospital. All the doctors live in the campus and do not practice privately as the code of hospital does not permit them. All the doctors of this hospital, some are from foreign also, provide their services on the very nominal salary — not on market prices.

In Vikasnagar there is one community health centre, which is over-crowded. Most of the serious cases referred to this hospital. In this hospital patients from all the sections of the society come, any concession, patient get on the assessment of the doctor. Hospital do not provide free of cost medicine, at least one rupee should be paid. This creates self-respect among poor-patients. For all the patients, medicines are provided from the hospital on subsidized rate. In the hospital, pathological lab facilities are also available.

'Christian Missionary Hospital' does not organize any health camp independently, but they sent their medical staff on the demand of any NGO, who organize health camps, like SMTA has organized eye camp which was lead by Missionary Hospital's doctors. They were operated in the Missionary Hospital at the free of cost. Lehman Hospital has started community health programme also. Their community health programme is running on the border of U.P. and Uttaranchal Pradesh in 'Badshai Bagh'. Under this programme adolescence related problems of literacy, immunization etc. come under it. Programme like 'Anugrah' is for the children who suffered from sexual abuse, get counseling on Sundays by psychologist of the hospital.

'Christian Missionary Hospital' is reliable in this area. Due to commitment, devotion, discipline and zeal to serve, of the staff, patients feel safe and satisfaction here. People have a praiseworthy opinion about this hospital. This Missionary Hospital is compensating the shortage and insufficient health-care facilities provided by the Govt. Health Care Institutions.

Case Study XII

Swajal Yojna (A joint venture of Govt. of India sponsored by World Bank to solve the problem of water supply)

Water is the most basic necessity for human health, and so is true for the people of Almora. But lack of this most basic necessity is making life most hard for the people of Almora. To solve this problem, the Government of India has started a project by the name of 'Swajal' with the aid from World Bank. **'Swajal'** means 'own water or water for the people of Almora from their own natural resources'. To save the people from the ill effects of lack of this basic necessity, Government of India has obtained projects from World Bank, worth millions of rupees and makes them self-reliant in water. This project is implemented in the villages for 2-3 yrs and when they become self-sufficient of water supply, it moves on to other places.

Swajal's main objective is to "save" water. In this process, water is saved in big tanks from many sources in the hills and taken to villages. There, the govt. spends 90% of the project cost and the rest 10% is collected in the form of share from the Villagers, as cash or labour. The maintenance and look after is left on the Villagers.

But this scheme is being moulded for their own benefit by some greedy organizations. As they make the scheme on paper, and contribution cough-up the regained 10% amount they arranged themselves, on behalf of villagers and then total amount distribute among them. In this way, Government of India and World Bank's scheme converted for them into a self-benefits scheme, and the money borrowed from World Bank is being returned in the form of interest from the hard earned money of the Indian masses, as the punishment of inefficiency of social schemes of the Government.

Since the look after of this scheme is left on villagers, it is not possible for them to look after the tanks and supplies of water, after the officials have left them on their own. There is nobody to help them.

The anomaly is where the govt. thinks that it has fulfilled its responsibility of providing water to the people, their problem remains as it is.

Bibliography

Abdul Kalam A.P.J. & **Rajan Y.S.** (1998) India Vision, 2020, Viking Penguin Books India (P) Ltd., New Delhi.

AcKrKnecht E.H. (1955), 'A Short History of Medicine', Ronalc Press, New York.

Adisehias, Malcolm (1989), 'Women, The Economic Discipline and the Labour Market', "Women and Development" by R.K. Sapru, Ashish Publishing House, Punjabi Bagh, New Delhi.

Agnihotri S.B. (2000), 'Sex Ratio Patterns in the Indian Population', Sage Publication, New Delhi, Thousand Oaks, London.

Agosin Marjorie (2003), 'Women Gender and Human Rights', A Global Perspective, Rawat Publication, Jaipur and New Delhi.

Alberecht G.L. and **Higgins P.C.** (1979), 'Health, Illness and Medicine, Chicago' Rand McNally College Publishing Company.

Altekar A.S. (1962), 'The Position of Women in Hindu Civilization' (From Pre-History to Present Day), IIIrd Edition, Moti Lal Banarsi Das, New Delhi.

Ammar H. (1960), 'The Sociologist Approach to Problem of Community Development', Sirsel Layyan, U.A.R., Arab States Fundamental Education Centre.

Anant Suchitra, Rao S.V.R. and Kapoor K. (1986), 'Women at Work, A Bibliography', Sage Publications, New Delhi.

Baig, Tara Ali (1976), 'Women Power of India', Sultanchand and Sons.

Bakshi, S.R. and **Bala Kiran** (1999), 'Development of Women, Children and Weaker Sections', Deep and Deep Publication Pvt. Ltd., New Delhi.

Bakshi, S.R. and **Bala Kiran** (2000), 'Welfare and Development of Women', Deep and Deep Publication Pvt. Ltd., N. Delhi.

Banerji (1995), 'Foundation for Research in Community Health', Newsletter IXth No. 1, Jan., Feb.

Banerji D. (1974), 'Social and Cultural Foundation of Health Services System', E.P.W. Vol. UX.

Banerji D. (1995), 'National Health Policy, its Implementation', Economic and Political Weekly, 22 Jan, pp. 105 - 108.

Banerji N. and **Jain D.** (1985), 'Tyrany of the House hold Women in Poverty', Shakti Books, Vikas Publishing House, New Delhi.

Banga, Ved Prakash (1996), 'Real Threat to Dignified Health Care,' New Delhi, Jai Medical Publication.

Baru (2002) Quoted in an article 'Medical Tourism' by Godwin S.K., E.P.W. Sept. 2004.

Berkman L.F. and **Syme S.L.** (1979), 'Social Networks, Host Resistance and Mortality', A Nine Year Follow-up of Alameda County Residents, American Journal of Epidemiology 109 : 186 - 204.

Bhandari Nita and **Supriya Mayank** (1999), 'A Study on Perceptions, Prevalence and Health Seeking Behaviour of Maternal Morbidities in a Urban Slum', Unpublished Report.

Bhatia J.C. (1972), 'Traditional Healer and Modern Medicine', SOC Sc. J.R. MED Vol. 19.

Bhowmick P.K. (1976), 'Socio-Cultural Profile of Frontier Bengal', Punthi Pustak.

Bhowmick P.K. and **Chaudry B.,** 'Some Aspects of Magico-Religious Beliefs and Practices of Mundas', Folklore, 8(3) 14 - 100.

Bhowmik P.K. (1955), 'Treatment of Disease among the Lodhas of West Bengal,' Man in India 1955, 35(4), 287 - 298.

Bodding P.O. (1925), 'The Santals and Disease', Memoirs of the A.S.B., Vol. 10, No. 1 pp. 1 - 127.

Brockington C.F. (1954), 'The Health of the Community', London, Churchile.

Brunner E. (1966), 'Health and Social Organization', Routledge, 11-New Fetter Lane, London.

Bunker J. (2001), 'Medicine Matters after all, In : Health and Disease' : A Reader, 3rd Edn. (eds. B. Davey, A. Gray & C. Seale), Open University, Buckingham.

Chadwic, E. (1842) (New Ed. 1965), 'Report on the Sanitary Conditions of Labouring Population of Great Britain', M. Flinn (ed) Edinburgh University Press.

Chapin, 'Experimental Designs : Sociological Research', pp. 28.

Chatterji M. (1993) 'Social Science and Health' (I.C.S.S.R.) 24 Jan. - March.

Chaudhari M.K. (2001) 'Health Policy, Strategy and Tribal Development in Tribal Health', Edited by Ramesh Chaubey and K.K.N. Sharma.

Chaudhari, B. (1986), 'Medical Anthropology in India with Special Reference to Tribal Population,' (In) "Tribal Health : Socio-Cultural Dimension" (Ed.) B. Chaudhuri Inter-India Publication, New Delhi.

Chaudhari, Renuka (2004), quoted in 'The Hindu', Chennai, June 8, 2004.

Chitnis Suma (1975), 'Significance of I.W.Y. for Women' 'Indian Women in Contemporary India', Edited by D. Souza, Manohar Book Service, Delhi, pp. 10 -19.

Clement, F.E. (1932) 'Primitive Concept of Disease', University of California Publications in American Archaeology Ethnology pp. 185 - 252.

Coe, R.M. (1978) 'Sociology of Medicine,' New York : McGraw, Hill Book Co.

Dandekar Kumudani (1957), 'A Demographic Survey of Rural Communities', in CSW Report (1974) Government of India Publication, New Delhi.

Dass, J.P. (1968), 'Authority, Power and Family Relationship in two Primitive Tribes of Orissa', The Eastern Anthropologist, Vol. XVI, No. 3.

David Blane, **Eric Brunner** and **Richard Wilkinson**, 'Health and Social Organization', Edited by Richard Wilkinson; London and New York.

David, B., Brunner, E., Wilkinson R. (1996), 'Health and Social Organization', Routledge 11, New Fetter Lane, London.

Davis and Black (1974), (Quoted in Report of the committee on the Status of Women in India) (1974).

Deminguel, Jesus M. (1979), 'A Framework for the study of National Health System' in Jaco, Gartly, E.A. Sources Book in Behaviour Sciences and Health, New York Press.

Desai (1998) Quoted in the Book, 'N.G.O.s : As Prime Movers', by Shivani Dharmrajan, Kaushik Publishers, Ansari Road, Daria Ganj, N. Delhi (2001).

Desai Neera (1957), 'Women in Modern India' (2nd Edition 1977), Vora and Co-Publishers, Bombay.

Desai Neera and **Krishan Raj Maitrye** (1987), 'Women and Society in India', Ajanta Publication, N. Delhi.

Desai Neera and **Patel Vibhuti** (1985), 'Indian Women : Change and Challenges in the International Decade 1975 - 1985', Popular Prakashan, Bombay.

Desai, M.D. (1966), 'Economic Life in a Rajasthan Village', Vallabh Vidyanagar, Sardar, Vallabhai Vidyapith, 1966.

Dharanrajan, Shivani (2001), 'N.G.O.s as Prime Movers', Kaushik Publishers Distributors, Ansari Road, Darya Ganj, New Delhi.

Dixon, M. (1979), 'Review of current Research on Health Nutrition and Medicine in Rural Alaska', Anthropological Association, Fair Banks, Alaska; in Ruffini, J.L. (ed) Advances in Medical Social Science, op. cit., (p. 218).

Djurfeldt, et al, **Goran** and **Lundberg** (1980), 'Pills against poverty : A Study in Tamil Villages', New Delhi, Mac Millan Company.

Dube Leela (2001), 'Anthropological Exploration in Gender Intersecting Fields', Sage Publications India Pvt. Ltd., M-32 Market, Greater Kailash - I, New Delhi.

Duggal Ravi, Sucheta Amin (1989), 'Cost of Health Care - A Household Survey in an Indian District', Mumbai.

Duraiswamy P.K. (1969), Swasth Hind, Vol. 13.

Durkhiem E. (1912), 'Le Suicide', New York; Free Press, pp. 246 - 252.

Durkheim E. (1938), 'The Rules of Sociological Method', Translated by Solovay S.A. and Mueller, J.H., Chicago : University of Chicago Press.

Durkheim, E. (1951) & (1952), 'Suicide : A Study in Sociology', New York Free Press.

Durkhiem E. (1893), 'Elementary Forms of Religious Life', New York; Free Press.

Eaton, J.W. (1958), 'Folk Obstertrics and Paediatrics Meet the M.D., A Case Study of Social Anthropology in Medicine', Patients, Physicians and Illness (ed.), E.G. Jaco Free, New York.

Elliott and Merril, 'Social Disorganization, p. 9.

Elwin V. (1942), 'A Maria Murder and Suicide', Oxford University Press, Bombay.

Elwin V. (1955), 'The Religion of an Indian Tribe', Oxford University Press, London.

Febrega H. Jr. and D.Silver (1970), 'Some Social and Psychological Properties of Zinaco Ntecoshaman, Behavioral Science Vol. 15, pp. 471 - 486.

Febrega, H. Jr. (1970), 'On the Speciricity of Folk Illnesses', South Western Journal of Anthropology Vol. 26, pp. 305 - 314.

Frake, C.O. (1961), 'The Diagnosis of Disease Among the Subanun of mind an as', American Anthropologists, Vol. 63, pp. 113 - 132.

Frank, J.D. (1961), 'Persuation and Healing, Johns Hopkins, Baltimore.

Friendson, E. (1967), 'Disability as Social Deviance', in Marvin, B. Sussman (ed) "Sociology and Rehabilitation," Washington, D.C. American Sociological Association, pp. 71 - 79.

Fuchs Stephen (1966), 'The Children of Hari : A Study of Nimar Balabis of Madhya Pradesh', Thacher and Co., Bombay.

Ghurye G.S. (1961), 'Class, Caste and Occupation', Bombay : Popular Book Depot.

Gillian Foo and Michael Koenig (2000), 'Quality of Care within the Indian Family Welfare Programme', In "Women's Reproductive Health in India" (ed.) by R. Ramasubban and Shireen J. Jejee Bhoy, Rawat Publication, Jaipur, New Delhi.

Godwin S.K. (2003, 2004), E.P.W.; Sept. 2004, 2003

Goffman, E (1990), 'Stigma : Notes on Management of Spoiled Identity', Penguin, London.

Goode & Hatt, 'Methods of Social Research', pp. 362.

Gopalan C. and Ramachandran P. (1989), 'Nutrition in Pregnancy', Women and Nutrition in India, New Delhi : Nutrition Foundation of India.

Gujral I.K.; 'An address by I.K. Gujral in a Science Congress at Hyderabad (1998), quoted in the 'India Vision 2020 by A.P.J. Abdul Kalam with Y.S. Rajan (1998), Viking Penguin Books, India.

Gupta (2004), E.P.W.; Sept, 2004.

Gupta Sunit, Mukta Gupta (1996, 2000), 'Role of Women in the Twenty First Century', Anmol Publication Pvt. Ltd., New Delhi.

Hassinger, E.W.Q. Report (Jan. 1958), L.M. "Relationships of the Public to Physicians in a Rural Setting." University of Missionary, Agricultural Experimental Station Research Bulletin, 653, 36.

Hema R. and **Murlidharan V.R.** (1983), 'Health and Human Resource Development', Economic and Political Weekly, Vol. XXVII, No. 43, October 23.

Hippocrates (1954), 'On Air, Water and Placs', in Ralph H. Major, A History of Medicine, Vol. I, Springfield : III Charles C. Thomas.

Howkins, N.G. (1950), 'Medical Sociology : Theory, Scope and Methods', Springfield, Illinosis, U.S.A. : Charles C. Thomas Publishers, pp. 3, 4 and 25.

Human Development Report (1993), U.N.D.P. Oxford University Press, p. 16.

I.C.S.S.R., I.C.M.R. Panel's Recommendation "A Decade Towards - Health For All".

Illich, I. (1990), 'Limits to Medicine, 'Medical Nemesis : The Expropriation of Health', Penguin, London.

Imboden, J.B. A.B. Center, L.E.Cliff and R.W. Trevo, R. (1961), "Symptomatic Recovery from Medical Disorders" Journal of American Medical Association, 178, pp. 1182 - 84.

Ishwaran, R. (1968) Sheopur : A South Indian Village "Rouledge and Kegonpaul".

Jarvis, D.S. (1958), 'Folk Medicine', Fawcett Greenwich Conn.

Jha, Jayawantha Rao (1954), Folkways Affecting Disease, Jabalpur.

Jill, C.H. and Geeta Menon (1994), Tribal Eco. Health.

Karna, M.N. (1981), 'Cast and Concept of Health in a North Bihar Village in Studies in Bihar's Economy and Society' by M.N. Karna (ed), Concept Publishing House, New Delhi.

Kellner, R.(1988), 'Physical Health, Mental Health and Excercise' in Appenzeller, O. (ed), Sports Medicine, Battimore Munich : Urban, pp. 73-84.

Khan, ME etal, (1989) Access to Health and Family Planning Services in Rural Uttar Pradesh; A Micro level evaluation, Journal of Family welfare, Vol. 35, No. 3 March pp. 3-20.

Khare, R.S. (1963), 'Folk Medicine in A North Indian Village', Human Organization, Vol. 22, No. 1.

Kidwai, M.H. Sheik (1978), "Women Under Different Social and Religious Laws', Life Publisher, New Delhi.

Koos, E.S. (1958), 'The Health of Regionville', Columbia University Press, New York, Brightmeer J. Ltd.

Kothari Gopa (1989), 'Woman's Health' in "Woman and Development" by R.K. Sapru, Ashish Publishing House, Punjabi Bagh, N. Delhi.

Krishn Raj, M. (1988), 'Women and Development : The Indian Experience', Shubhadra and Saraswati Prakashan, Pune.

Kroeger, A. (1980), 'Housing and Health in the Process of Cultural Adaptation : A Case Study among Jungle and High Land Natives of Ecuador', Journal of Tropical Medicine and Hygiene, Vol. 83, pp. 53 - 69.

Kumar S. Vijaya and **Chakrapani C.** (1995), 'Availability, Accessibility and Utilisation of Rural Health and Services', The Journal of Family Welfare, Vol. 41(3), September.

Kumar, A.K. (2004) 'Frontline' December 4 (2004).

Kumar, Ashok (1990), 'Development, Women and Children in India', Common Wealth Publishers, Ansari Road, N. Delhi.

Le Famu. J. (1999) 'The Rise and Fall of Modern Medicine', Little Brown & Co., London.

Lewis, Oscar, 'Village life in Northern India', New York Random House, Ine.

Linton Ralf "The cultural Background of Personality" p. 264.

Madan, T.N. (1980), Doctors and Society, New Delhi : Vikas Publishing House Pvt. Ltd.

Majumdar Veena, (1978) 'Symbols of Power,' SNDT University Bombay Allied Publishers.

Marriott, M, (1955), 'Western Medicine in a village of North India, Health in Culture and Community,' B.D. Paul (ed) Russel Sage, New York, pp. 252-253.

Marx K. (1964), 'Selected Writing in Sociology and Social Philosophy,' translated by T.B. Bottomore, London, Mc Graw- Hill pp. 51-78.

Mathew, P.M., Nair M.S. (1986), 'Women Organisations.' Ashish Publishing House, New Delhi pp. 1-14.

Mathews, C.M.E. (1979) 'Health and Culture in A South Indian Village', New Delhi: Sterling Publishers.

Mckeown, T. (1979) 'The role of Medicine, 'Blachwell, Oxford.

Mehta S.R. (1987) 'Aspects of health and illness', The Journal of Sociological Studies, Vol. 16, January.

Mehta Usha, Aggarwal Alka (2000), 'Hygeine first Aid and home nursing.

Meiss Maria (1980) 'Indian Women and Patriarchy' - Concept, New Delhi.

Milan L.C. (1974), 'Ethnohistory of Disease and Medical Care among the Aleut.' Anthropological Papers of the University of Alaska. 16(2); 15-40.

Miner, L, (1956) 'The Body Ritual of the Nacireme', American Anthropologists, Vol. 58, June pp. 503-507.

Ministry of Health (Govt. of India) 1983, 'The National Policy of Health.'

Morris, J.N., (1973) 'Four Cheers for Prevention', Pro. Roy. soc. Med. vol 66:225.

Mukherjee, Prabhati (1978) 'Hindu women Normative Models, Orient Longman Lib. New Delhi.

Muraleedharan, V.R (1993) 'When is Access to Health Care Equal', Some public policy issues,' Economic and Political Weekly, 28 (25) 19 June, pp. 129-196.

Muraleedhraran, V.R. (1979), 'Rural Health care in Madras Presidency', The Indian Economic and Social Review, Vol. 24, no, 3.

Nagla Madhu (1997) "Sociology of Medical Profession", Prem Rawat for Rawat Publications, 3-Na-20, Jawahar Nagar, Jaipur 302004, India.

Nagraj K.N. (2006) "The Hindu" January 4 (2006).

Netting R.M. (1973) 'Fighting Forest and Fly : Some Demographic regulators among the Katyar' Journal of Anthropological Research, Vol. 29, No. Aug. pp. 164-179.

Newman, P.L. (1964) 'Wildman Behaviour in a New Guinea High Land Community.' American Anthopologist Vol. 66 pp. 1-19.

Nyammathi, A. Leake, B. Keehan, C. Gulberg, L. (2000) 'Type of social support among homeless women : Its impact on Psychosocial Resources,' Health and health behaviour and use of services. Nursing Research 49, 316-326.

Ogburn W.F. (1972). 'A Hand Book of Sociology,' New Delhi, Eurasia Publishing House Pvt. Ltd. p. 257.

Opler, M.E. 91963. 'The Cultural Definition of Illness in village India.' Human organisation Vol. 22 No. 1.

Pandey Mrinal (2006), 'जनस्वास्थ्य सुविधाओं की षवसाधना', हिन्दुस्तान, जनवरी 15] 2006.

Paranjape, Sarina (1989) 'Women's Educational Status' in "Women and Development," by R.K. Sapru, Aashish Publishing House, Punjabi Bagh, New Delhi.

Parsons, T (1951), 'The Social System', New York Free Press, pp. 428-473.

Parsons, T (1972), 'Definition of Health and Illness in the Light of American Values and Social Structure,' in E.G. Jaco (ed) "Patient, Physicians and Illness," New York. Free Press pp. 107.

Planning Commission (1996), Ninth Five Year Plan, 1997-2002, Vol. New Delhi, Government of India.

Pokrana K.L. (1994) 'Social Beliefs, Cultural Practices in Health and Diseases,' Rawat publication, Jaipur and New Dehi.

Qadeer, Imrana, (1998) 'Reproductive Health - A Public Health Perspective,' E.P.W., Vol. XXXIII, No. 41, Oct. 10-6.

Radcliff-Brown A.R. (1940) 'Introduction in African System of Kinship and Marriage' (ed) London, Oxford University Press.

Radcliffe- Brown (1971) 'Structure and Function in Primitive Society', in Coser and Rosenborg in "Sociological Theory" (eds) R. Brown, New York, McMillan.

Ramasubbam R. and Jejee Bhoy J. Shreen (2000) 'Women's Reproductive Health in India', Rawat Publication, Satyam Apartments, Sector-3, Jawahar Nagar, Jaipur.

Ramchandran, L. and Dharmalinghm T. (1983) 'Text Book of Health Education,' New Delhi, Vikas Publishers, pp. 103-104.

Rao. P.S.S. 'Study on Socio-economic and Demographic Correlates of Medical Care Utilisation and Health Behaviour' Research Report, Indian Council of Social Science Research, New Delhi.

Reissman C.K. (1974) 'The Use of Health Services by the Poor.', Social Policy Vol. 5, no. 1, May June, pp. 41 - 49.

Rishyasringa B. and Ramasubbam R. (2000), 'Treatment Seeking by Women in Mumbai Slums', paper presented at a Workshop on Reproductive Health in India, New Evidence and Issues, Pune, March.

Roemer, M.I. (1976) 'A Rural Health Care,' St. Luise C.V. Musby.

Roy, M. (1985) 'Primary Health Care in India' Health and Population Perspective and Issues, Vol. 8, No. 3.

Sachidananda, (1986, 1994), 'Socio-Cultural Dimensions of Tribal Health', Journal of Social and Economic Studies, New Series 3-4 , Oct-Dec., pp. 389-401.

Sainath, P., (2006), 'The Hindu', Jan. 4, 2006.

Shrinivasan, V., (2001); 'Health and Family Welfare Programmes in Developing Countries' Allekh Publishers, Dugger Building, M.I. Road, Jaipur.

Samuel, S.A. (1989), 'Women's Health and Role in Population Education', in "Woman and Development" by R.K. Sapru, Ashish Publishing House, Punjabi Bagh, New Delhi.

Sapru ,R.K; (1989), 'Woman and Development,' Ashish Publishing House, Punjabi Bagh, New Delhi.

Saunder S.L (1954) 'Cultural Difference and Medical Care', Russell Sage Foundation, New York pp. 144-145

Saunder, J.V.D. & H. Bruening, (1959) 'Hospital Community Relations in Mississippi,' Rural Sociology, 24 March, pp. 48-51.

Shanthi K., (1998), "Empowerment of Women" ; Professor, Department of Econometrics and Coordinator Centre for Gender Studies, University of Madras, Chennai.

Sharma, O.P. (2000) "Rural Health and Medical Care in India", Manak Publication, G-19, Vijay Chok Laxmi Nager New Delhi.

Shattuck L. (1948) 'Report of the Sanitary Commission of Massachusetts,' 1850, Cambridge M.A., Harward University Press.

Shaver LG, (1982), Essentials of Exercise Physiology, Delhi, Surjeet Publication, pp. 168-195.

Sigerist, H.E. (1951) 'A History of Medicine,' Vol. 1, Oxford University Press Fair, London, N.J.

Singh, Jaswant, (2003), quoted in 'The Financial Times', July-2-2003.

Singh, S, Srivastava S.P., (2001), 'Gender Equality Through Women's Empowerment', Bharat Book Centre, Ashok Marg, Lucknow.

Singh, Shiv Raj, (1989), 'Woman and Rural Development in Hills', "Woman and Development" (Edited) by R.K. Sapru, Ashish Publishing House, Punjabi Bagh, New Delhi.

Sinha, R.K. (1951), 'Structure of Lower Class Families in Lucknow', Doctoral Dissertation, University of Lucknow.

Sorokin, P.A. (1951), 'Social and Cultural Mobility, Glenes Free Press.

Spencer, H. - ' The Principals of Sociology'.

Sri Devi, C, (1989) "Woman, Family, Health and Folk Medicine", Woman and Development by R.K. Sapru, Ashish Publishing House, Punjabi Bagh, New Delhi.

Srinivasan (1987), 'Management of Rural Health Care', Social Change, March, Vol. 17, No.1, pp. 24-33.

Srinivasan . S; (1987), "Management of Rural Health Care', Social Change, Vol. 17, No.1 March.

Stevenson L. (1975), 'The Belief and Cases Related to Reincarnation among the Haida', Journal of Anthropological Research, Vol. - 31, No. 4, Win., pp. 364-375.

Sujatha V. (2003), 'Health by the People : Sociology of Medical Lore', Rawat Publication, Jaipur and New Delhi.

Swain, S.A., Agarwal K., Ojha and A Prakash, (1994), "Determinants of Maternal Mortality : A Hospital Based from North India", Journal of Obstetrics and Gynaecology of India, 44.

Szreter, S. (1988) , 'The Importance of Social Intervention in Britain and Mortality Decline,' Social History of Medicine 1, 1-38.

Taylor, S. and David Field, 'Sociology of Health and Healthcare', Blackwell & Publishing, U.S.A.

'The Hindu' , January -4, (2006), A Survey by Hindu (2006).

'The Hindu' December- 28 (2005),

'Towards Equality: Report of the Commission for the Status of Woman in India', (C.S.W.I. 1974), Publication of Government of India, Ministry of Education and Social Welfare, Department of Social Welfare, New Delhi. (December 1974)

UNESCO Report, (1983).

United Nations (U.N.), (1994), 'Population and Development: Programme of Action Adopted at the International Conference on Population and Development,' Cairo Section -12, 17, ST/ESR.A/149, New York.

United Nations Human Development Report, (2005)

Vaidyanathan, K.E. (1972), (Ed), 'Mortality in India', Madurai, (Quoted from, The Report of C.S.W.I 1974 Govt. of India Publication).

Venkatesh Srinivasan, (1987), 'Health and Family Welfare Programmes in Developing Countries', Published Under the Auspices of the Centre for Administrative Change.

Vidyarthi, L.P. (1974), Tribal Development in Independent India and its Future, 'Man in India' Vol. 54, No. 1, Jan-Mar, pp. 45-72.

Visaria, L. (2000), 'From Contraceptive Targets to Informed Choice: The Indian Experience', in "Women's Reproductive Health in India" by Ramashubham and Shireen Jejeebhoj, Rawat Publications, Jaipur and New Delhi.

Visaria, L., (1998), 'The Quality of Reproductive Health Care in Gujarat: Perspectives of Female Health Workers and their Clients', In M.A. Koenig and M.K. Khan (eds), Improving Quality of Care in India's Family Welfare Programme : The Challenge Ahead, pp. 143-68. New York: The Population Council.

Weber Max, (1964), 'The Theory of Social and Economic Organization', Glencoe; Free Press.

Weber Max., (1906), 'Protestant Ethics and Sprit of Capitalism'

Whipple (2001), Quoted in "आर्थिक विकास और नियोजन" by M.P. Singh.

WHO Report (1947), 1948, 1978, 1987.

World Health Organisation (WHO), (1997) 'Unsafe Abortion: Global and Regional Estimates of Incidence and Mortality due to Unsafe Abortion with a Listing of Available Country Data', Division of Reproductive Health WHO/RHT/MSM/ 97.16 , Geneva : WHO.

Yadav, M.S., (1994) 'आदिवासी समुदाय में स्वास्थ्य के कुछ पक्ष', Rawat Publication, 3-Na-20,Jawahar Nagar, Jaipur 302004, India.

यजुर्वेद, 36/24.

Yesudian (1981), 'Differential Utilization of Health'.

Young, K. (1957), "Hand Book of Social Psychology", London : Routledge and Kegan Paul Ltd., p. 187.

Index

G

H

I

J

V

W